DIABETES IN THE REAL WORLD

DIABETES IN THE REAL WORLD

Charles Fox

Consultant Physician with Special Interest in Diabetes, Northampton General Hospital Trust

Anthony Pickering

General Practitioner, Northamptonshire

CLASS PUBLISHING · LONDON

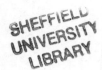
© Charles Fox, Anthony Pickering 1995

The rights of Charles Fox and Anthony Pickering to be identified as the authors of this work have been asserted by them in accordance with the Copyright, Designs and Patents Act 1988

Printing history
First published 1995

The authors and publishers welcome feedback from the users of this book. Please contact the publishers:
Class Publishing (London) Ltd.,
7 Melrose Terrace, London W6 7RL, UK.
Tel: 0171 371 2119
Fax: 0171 371 2878 [International +4471]

A CIP catalogue record for this book is available from the British Library

ISBN   1 872362 53 2

Designed by Florencetype Ltd, Stoodleigh, Devon
Edited by Richenda Milton-Thompson
Typeset by Florencetype Ltd, Stoodleigh, Devon
Production by Landmark Production Consultants Ltd, Princes Risborough

Printed and bound in Great Britain by
Clays Ltd, St Ives plc

CONTENTS

Part IV   Education

Appendices

ACKNOWLEDGEMENTS

We would like to thank our colleagues in Northampton, in particular Anne Kilvert and Jo Anthony for their advice about diabetic pregnancy and permission to reproduce the Northampton Guidelines on Gestational Diabetes. Also, John O'Donnell for help with lipids, and Kate Lindenbaum and Brian Hopkisson for suggestions about eye disease.

We have bounced most of our ideas off other members of the Northampton diabetes team – specialist nurses Maureen Brewin, Elaine Waring and Jan Anfield, and podiatrist Julie Mason.

Our approach to diabetes care has been shaped by Chris Gillespie, Suzanne Redmond, Florence Brown and many others who take part in the Northampton Diabetes Counselling Course.

We thank Robert Turner of the Diabetes Research Laboratories, Oxford, for permission to quote results of the UK Prospective Diabetes Study.

Throughout the task of writing, we have dipped frequently into three excellent textbooks: *Diabetes: Clinical Management* by Robert Tattersall and Edwin Gale (Longman, 1990) the *International Textbook of Diabetes Mellitus* by Alberti, DeFronzo, Keen and Zimmet (John Wiley, 1992) and the *Textbook of Diabetes* by John Pickup and Gareth Williams (Blackwell Science, 1991).

Peter Sönksen and Sue Judd have kindly allowed us to reproduce or adapt material from the third edition of *Diabetes at Your*

Fingertips (Class Publishing, 1994), namely Figures 4.3, 7.1, 7.2 and 9.1, the questions and answers featured in Chapter 18, and the 'Patient-friendly glossary' from Appendix 2.

Michael Loudon and Tom Humphries have put a huge amount of energy and skill into correcting and polishing the text. Kay Wright compiled the index and Carrie Walker read the proofs.

Richard Warner encouraged us to embark on this project and Richenda Milton-Thompson worked late into the night to pull our ideas into some semblance of order.

Novo-Nordisk, without whose support none of this would have been posible, and Professor Eva Kohner gave permission for use of the colour plates featured in this book. Novo-Nordisk also supplied the Insulin Chart from which Figure 5.1 has been adapted.

Finally, we pay tribute to our patients for helping us to understand what their lives are like and for giving us an insight into the real world of diabetes.

Charles Fox
Tony Pickering

INTRODUCTION

DAY TO DAY
DIABETES

"The author is living in cloud cuckoo land — what about the real world?"

Is this sentiment familiar? It can arise because of a conflict between the intellect and the emotion. The one is keen to learn, the other is responding to a reflection about practice in the real world.

In this book, we try to feed the intellect without leaving the bitter taste of inadequacy or anger. We attempt to deal with some of the problems and issues of diabetes from the perspective of people at the coal face. The authors are a consultant physician with an interest in diabetes, working in a district general hospital, and a general practitioner.

Diabetes in the Real World is about a few facts and lots of dilemmas, a small amount of "should" and a considerable helping of "try". It is an attempt to offer ideas about managing real problems in a world characterised by imperfections and uncertainty.

If medicine might be regarded as a cocktail of truths, half truths and downright prejudice, diabetes is a prime example. There are two complex variables at work: the *patient* with his or her particular make-up (both psychological and physiological), and the *condition*. Until recently a third variable, that there had been little research upon which to base our advice, further compounded the problem. We had followed a path of maximal, theoretical, potential gain for minimal anticipated cost. For example, if it turns out to be true that good glycaemic control prevents complications, then the penalty of failure is far greater than the cost of adherence. At least now some of our advice can be justified. It remains the case, however, that belief and knowledge may be confused, that much is not known, and that any individual health professional may not know all that is known. In addition, the workers of the Cochrane Institute at Oxford have demonstrated that it can take up to ten years for sound behaviours, evidence-based medicine, to become accepted in the medical culture. Furthermore, have we not all encountered patients who are resistant to change? Finally, this situation is compounded by an expectation from some patients that professionals will provide all the answers to their problems.

In this book we have attempted, in the "Commandments", to make firm recommendations based on information which is as near certain as possible. The remaining content comprises simple opinion, to be considered and debated, and views supported by "soft" evidence or logic of a sort. Much of the text, therefore, is offered for contemplation − as suggestion rather than as truth.

References are not cited in this book and this is deliberate. We are not attempting a scholarly or complete description of all aspects of diabetes. We do not want to distract the reader's attention by repeated references to other works.

The text may lack style in some parts. We have even tried to be humorous on occasion. We make no apology for either of these characteristics. This is how we, the authors, communicate − in official correspondence, socially, or to colleagues. We write as we live, between friends, each with particular interests, skills and problems, in the real world.

We use the device of letters, questions from a GP and answers from a specialist, to illustrate some of the dilemmas and offer an approach to dealing with the problems. Some are contrived; others are based on real cases. If the reader disagrees with a view expressed, so much the better. We will have provoked reflection and stimulated a search for information. We would welcome opinion on the views we express and will reply to any reader who writes to our publisher.

In writing this book we have had certain principles in mind:

■ **The concept of certainty**
We believe that, in medicine, certainty is more of a relative probability and, as such, is liable to change as new information accrues

■ **The rights of patients**
- To control their own lives and to make informed decisions which, occasionally, may damage their health
- To be treated as adults and, if they wish, as partners
- To the best treatment we can offer

(The corollary is that they, not the professionals, are responsible for their health)

■ **The role of the professional in chronic disease**
- As adviser and, if possible, partner
- We are consulted because of our knowledge and objectivity

■ **Education**
- Education is a continuing process, for us and for our patients
- We can learn from each other
- Both parties need to be questioning and flexible

Diabetes care invites humility and collaboration. Most of us have made a suggestion in good faith, based on experience, belief or logic, only to discover in the next consultation that it was a mistake. The whole culture of diabetes education is based on collaboration, as evidenced by the founding of the British Diabetic Association by two eminent people with diabetes (the author HG Wells and the doctor RD Lawrence). They wrote to *The Times* in 1934 to set up "An Association open to all diabetics, rich or poor, for mutual aid and assistance and to promote the study, the diffusion of knowledge, and the proper treatment of diabetes in this country". We have tried to foster the notion of collaboration, working out solutions with our patients.

We invite the reader, with these assertions in mind, to amble through this book and think about how the matters we discuss relate to him or her, to real patients, and the real world.

WHAT IS DIABETES?

2

The practice nurse pops her head round the door of your consulting room – Jim Brown has got sugar in his urine. "Yes OK. Why don't you measure his blood sugar?" (Nowadays nearly every practice nurse has the use of a blood glucose meter.) "I've done that and it's 18" is the reply. The ball is now in your court. What to do next? Should you panic? Eighteen sounds a bit too high for comfort.

By the time Jim is sitting down in your consulting room, he will be feeling alarmed and may have picked up the dreaded word DIABETES. As he sits down, ask yourself the following questions:

■ Is Jim fat?
■ Is he young or middle-aged plus?
■ Is he looking slightly ill, or perhaps very ill?

Ask your nurse whether she has tested his urine for ketones. If she has thrown away the sample, does his breath smell of ketones (pear drops)? Has he been vomiting?

Ask Jim how he feels. Is he thirsty? Has he been peeing a lot, feeling weak, or itchy "down below"? Has he lost any weight recently? And how long has he had these symptoms?

Take a brief family history, concentrating on diabetes and any bad effects it had on anyone.

Ask Jim what he, himself, knows about diabetes.

PANIC (EARLY REFERRAL TO A SPECIALIST) IF:

- Jim is young (under 30) and thin
- He has lost a lot of weight
- He has ketones in his urine, or on his breath
- He has been vomiting
- He has sighing respiration and is drowsy
- He feels weak and very unwell

RELAX IF:

- Jim is older
- He is fat
- He feels well, apart from a bit of thirst
- He has no ketones

These are, of course, the characteristics of insulin and non-insulin dependent diabetes (see Figure 2.1). Throughout this book we will use the following convention:

IDDM   Insulin dependent diabetes mellitus
IDD   Insulin dependent diabetic (the person with IDDM)
NIDDM   Non-insulin dependent diabetes mellitus
NIDD   Non-insulin dependent diabetic (the person with NIDDM)

The diagnosis of diabetes is not to be taken lightly but it can usually be made without the need for a glucose tolerance test (GTT). A random plasma glucose greater than 11 mmol/l, plus the typical symptoms, secures the diagnosis. If the random glucose is less than 11 mmol/l, the next step is to arrange a plasma glucose measurement after an overnight fast. Since the diagnosis is so important, it is worth sending a sample to the laboratory and not relying on the surgery blood glucose meter. A fasting plasma glucose greater than 8 mmol/l confirms the diagnosis. In the rare cases where the fasting glucose is below 8 mmol/l, a GTT is needed. This can be done by giving 75 g glucose by mouth after an overnight fast, taking

Figure 2.1

Comparison of insulin dependent (IDDM) and non-insulin dependent diabetes mellitus (NIDDM)

	IDDM	NIDDM
Alternative names	TYPE I	TYPE II
	juvenile onset	maturity onset
Treatment	insulin	diet and/or tablets
		and/or insulin
Age of onset	less than 30 yrs	middle-aged
Overweight	no	yes
Ketones	yes	no
Genetic link	strong	very strong
Autoimmune disease	yes	no

Figure 2.2

Oral 75 g glucose tolerance test (GTT). Diagnostic criteria

	Glucose concentration in mmol/l			
	Plasma		Whole blood	
	Venous	Capillary	Venous	Capillary
Diabetes mellitus				
fasting value	≥7.8	≥7.8	≥6.7	≥6.7
or 2-hour value	≥11.1	≥12.2	≥10.0	≥11.1
Impaired glucose tolerance				
fasting value	≥7.8	≥7.8	≥6.7	≥6.7
or 2-hour value	7.8–11.1	8.9–12.2	6.7–10.0	7.8–11.1

samples before and two hours after the glucose load. The WHO guidelines, published in 1985, for interpreting GTTs are shown in Figure 2.2.

INITIAL TREATMENT

What does "dependent" actually mean?

Diabetes has for years been divided into insulin dependent diabetes (mellitus) – IDDM for short – and non-insulin dependent diabetes or NIDDM. These unwieldy terms are meant to be helpful in distinguishing the two main types of diabetes but they can be confusing. People with IDDM are literally *dependent* on insulin and, if deprived of it, their blood glucose level will rise and they will start breaking down their body fat to produce ketones. These biochemical acids cause metabolic mayhem, leading to coma and death. This process can only be prevented by giving insulin.

On the other hand the term NIDDM does not say anything about the treatment the patient may need. The majority achieve good control on diet alone at the outset. After a time tablets are needed to maintain a relatively normal blood glucose, and a significant proportion end up on insulin. Thus there are many NIDDs who are insulin-treated diabetics.

The differences between the two main types of diabetes go much deeper than simply age of onset and the shape of the patient.

Genetics

The two types of diabetes have different genetics, with IDDM associated with certain tissue typing (HLA) antigens. The closest association has been found with DR3 and DR4 and if someone carries both these antigens they have a 20 times greater risk of developing IDDM than a person without either of these markers. Thus there is strong evidence that the development of IDDM is genetically determined, and one might guess that in NIDDM the genetic links are weaker. However, studies on identical twins have shown the opposite to be true. If one of a pair of identical twins has IDDM, there is a 30-50% chance that the other twin will have IDDM. However, it is the rule that if one twin has NIDDM, then *both* twins will. In other words, concordance for IDDM is less than 50%, while that for NIDDM is 100%.

Immunity

In addition to the genetic link, IDDM is an autoimmune disease. The best evidence for this is that antibodies to islet cells in the pancreas are usually present in people who are developing IDDM. There is a study in progress which examines closely the relatives of children who have IDDM. If high titres of islet cell antibodies appear in the blood of any of the siblings, it is likely that they will develop IDDM themselves. By the time the insulin producing beta cells have been destroyed and the patient has diabetes, the islet cell antibodies have often disappeared from the blood.

Further evidence that immunity and genetics play a part in IDDM comes from the fact that patients with IDDM and their families are at greater risk of other autoimmune diseases such as Graves' disease of the thyroid, pernicious anaemia, vitiligo and Addison's disease. These associations do not apply to NIDDM and there is no evidence that immune mechanisms are involved in this type of diabetes.

OTHER TYPES OF DIABETES

Most of these are rare in the community. They need to be considered whenever the clinical presentation is unusual, and are listed in Figure 2.3.

The following causes of diabetes are not uncommon in a hospital-based diabetic clinic.

Figure 2.3 Causes of secondary diabetes

Pancreatic
> Chronic pancreatitis
> Carcinoma of the pancreas
> Cystic fibrosis
> Haemochromatosis

Hormonal
> Cushing's syndrome
> Thyrotoxicosis
> Acromegaly

Drug-induced
> Steroids
> Thiazide diuretics

Rare genetic syndromes
> Prader-Willi syndrome
> Freidrich's ataxia
> DIDMOAD (diabetes insipidus, diabetes mellitus, optic atrophy, deafness)

Maturity onset diabetes of the young (MODY)

Steroid induced

This is found in patients receiving long-term steroids for rheumatoid arthritis and asthma. It should be treated in the normal way, with diet first, followed by tablets and, if necessary, insulin. The treatment needed to control diabetes may be very sensitive to the dose of steroids and it can be frustrating for the patient and diabetologist if the dose of steroids is constantly altered around the threshold at which insulin is required.

People with tablet-controlled diabetes under care of oncologists may be given very large doses of steroids for up to ten days on a cyclical basis. These patients should check their blood glucose carefully and if it reaches the high teens and they feel thirsty, it is best to give them insulin for the duration of the steroid arm of the cycle.

People who are terminally ill are often given dexamethasone to perk them up. This can be helpful but every so often leads to diabetes which does not respond to oral hypoglycaemics. If it can be shown that dexamethasone really improves the quality of life, at the same time as the raised sugar levels are making the patient dry, insulin may need to be given. It is important to be therapeutically imaginative in terminal care, and to ask the patient to take part in the process of making decisions.

Chronic pancreatitis

This is a common cause of diabetes. It may be associated with the added complication of exocrine pancreatic failure, leading to the need for replacement of pancreatic enzymes in the form of Pancrex or Creon. Worse still, these patients may lack glucagon, an important component of the counter-regulatory response to hypoglycaemia. Metabolic control may be hampered by malabsorption and extra sensitivity to insulin.

Cancer of the pancreas

This usually presents with progressive weight loss, abdominal pain and, sometimes, jaundice. Occasionally a patient may present as a routine NIDD and initially lose weight very successfully in response to dieting. Only when the weight loss continues and there is pain in the abdomen and back is the true diagnosis suspected. At this stage an abdominal ultrasound is the first line investigation to look for pancreatic malignancy.

CONTROL

3

Good control means different things to different people. To the person with diabetes, it means being able to live a normal life. To the carer it means the absence of hypoglycaemic episodes (hypos). To the diabetes specialist it means maintenance of the best possible blood glucose levels, which is reflected in levels of glycosylated haemoglobin (HbA1c) in the acceptable range.

Is good control important?

This has been the unanswered question haunting diabetes care since it was first discovered that insulin therapy did not prevent the long term complications of diabetes. There have been many attempts to investigate the relationship between control and complications, including both animal experiments and a large retrospective survey of 4400 patients in Belgium. Over the past ten years a number of prospective studies were carried out in Scandinavia. These indicate that tight metabolic control at least slows the progress of complications.

The Diabetes Control and Complications Trial (DCCT)

This study, the most definitive to date, came out of North America and quantified the reduction in microvascular disease achievable by good control of blood glucose. The problem with describing the DCCT is that it was really two studies in one. The first component looked at the effect of "tight" versus "normal" control in a group of 726 patients free from any detectable complications (the Primary Prevention group). The second component (Secondary Intervention) consisted of a group of 715 patients who had already developed early but measurable complications due to the typical small vessel disease caused by diabetes. Each group was randomly allocated to either intensive ("tight") or conventional ("normal") therapy. The success of the study lay in the remarkable adherence to the designated metabolic status achieved particularly by the "tight" control group.

The DCCT continued for nine years, and throughout this period, patients in the "tight" control group maintained a mean HbA1c which never exceeded 7.1%. Mean HbA1c in the conventionally treated group was 9%.

The two principal questions addressed were:

■ Would "tight" control in the Primary Prevention group prevent the development and subsequent progression of retinopathy?

■ Would "tight" control in the Secondary Intervention group affect the progression of retinopathy?

Patients in both groups were randomised to receive either conventional therapy (with one or two insulin injections per day) or intensive therapy (administered either by external insulin pump or by three or more daily insulin injections together with frequent blood glucose monitoring), and closer, more regular contact with their health care professionals. Ninety-seven per cent of subjects complied with the treatment regimen to which they were assigned.

The patients were followed for between three and nine years

Figure 3.1

Benefits of intensive treatment

	Primary prevention	Secondary intervention
Retinopathy	76% less*	54% less*
Microalbuminuria	34% less*	43% less*
Albuminuria	—	56% less*
Neuropathy	69% less*	57% less*

Indicates percentage reduction in complication compared with conventional control

(mean 6.5 years), during which the progression of complications was assessed regularly. The benefits enjoyed by those with intensive treatment are shown in Figure 3.1.

Although intensive therapy was effective, both in delaying the onset and in slowing the progression of retinopathy, nephropathy and neuropathy in patients with IDDM, "tight" control was also found to increase some risks of diabetes care – as shown in Figure 3.2.

Figure 3.2

Costs of tight control

	Intensive treatment	Conventional treatment
Severe hypos per 100 patient years	62	19
Coma per 100 pt years	16	5
Fatal road traffic accident	2	1
Hospitalisation (for hypo)	54	36
Obesity	12.7	9.3

Limitations of the DCCT results

Patients who took part in the DCCT were not simply the next 1500 people with diabetes who happened to present to the participating clinics. They were very carefully selected for the trial after stringent practical and psychological tests intended to ensure that they would endure the constraints of the study.

No expense was spared in the support of those patients in the intensive control group. They kept in close contact with their medical attendants throughout the duration of the study, which averaged 6.5 years. It has been calculated that investing to this level in the UK would cost an extra £720 per patient per year.

Because the average age of the participants in the DCCT was only 27 years, and large vessel disease is rare in this age group, the total score of large vessel disease was less than one event per 100 patient years, a number insufficient for the detection of significant differences.

Patients' experience of the DCCT

The message of the DCCT is a stark one. The struggle to achieve tight control significantly reduces the risk of complications but carries an increased likelihood of severe hypos. Patients might feel threatened by this newly defined dilemma, but when the DCCT is discussed – either in groups or individually – most patients give the impression that they are already only too aware of their predicament. The detailed statistics do not cut much ice with patients; they are not usually interested in chances or risks but understandably want to know whether they are going to be one of the lucky or the unlucky ones.

At the collective level, the British Diabetic Association organised a meeting of patients and professionals "to explore the implications of the DCCT on diabetes management in the UK".

The group came up with three broad recommendations:

■ The DCCT *must not* be used as a stick to bully people living with diabetes into meeting clinical targets.

■ It should be used to influence the Department of Health, NHS Trusts and District Health Authorities to improve services to patients. There is a clear need for more resources.

■ People working in diabetes care need to put more emphasis on treating each person living with diabetes, both holistically and as an individual.

Out of this group has grown the Better Care Action Group which aims by information to encourage people with diabetes to become more actively involved in their own care and to improve the knowledge, attitudes and skills of health care professionals.

The UKPDS (control in NIDDM)

While the effects of intensive treatment of patients with IDDM have been shown by the DCCT, the United Kingdom Prospective Diabetes Study (UKPDS), currently in progress, is examining the effects of different treatment regimens in patients with NIDDM. This study was piloted in six centres in 1977 and now includes 5102 patients in 23 centres in England, Scotland and Northern Ireland. After a four-month period on diet alone, patients with a fasting plasma glucose greater than 6 mmol/l were randomised to either continuing on diet alone or to treatment with sulphonylureas or insulin. Patients who were obese could also be randomised to metformin therapy.

Following randomisation and stabilisation of treatment, patients are seen every three or four months and receive a programme of routine clinical assessment and care which is detailed in Figure 3.3.

Figure 3.3

UKPDS routine clinical care/assessment

Every three months	Fasting plasma glucose
	Body weight
	Blood pressure
	Dietary advice
	Change in therapy
	Reporting side-effects
Annually	*As above plus*
	HbA1c
	Biochemistry
	Visual acuity
	Retinal screening
	Foot examination
	Health questionnaire
Three-yearly	*As above plus*
	Routine bloods
	Chest X-ray
	ECG
	Retinal photography
	Biosthesiometer (vibration threshold)
	Doppler studies

Results of the UKPDS

Unlike the DCCT, which recruited an unusual type of IDD into the study, patients in the UKPDS are a representative cross-section of people with NIDDM from the UK.

The study is scheduled to finish in 1998, when the relative benefit of the various treatments will be revealed. The careful monitoring of UKPDS patients has already shown that hypos are surprisingly common in those taking glibenclamide and chlorpropamide, and that metformin is effective in reducing

Figure 3.4

Complications of diabetes occuring by 1993 among all patients participating in the UKPDS

	Percentage
Macrovascular complications	
Myocardial infarction	8.9
(including sudden death)	
Angina and abnormal ECG	4.4
Heart failure	1.9
Stroke	2.8
Any macrovascular end-point	15.4
Microvascular complications	
Need for retinal photocoagulation	5.0
Vitreous haemorrhage	0.4
Blindness	2.0
Renal failure	0.5
Any microvascular clinical end-point	6.4

plasma glucose without leading to an increase in body weight. It has also highlighted the additional risk incurred by patients with both diabetes *and* hypertension. Follow-up so far has shown that hypertension is associated with a twofold risk of heart attack and a threefold risk of stroke and amputation, compared with normotensive NIDDs. In contrast, hypertension seems to have little or no effect on the risk of small vessel disease such as retinopathy.

The overall complication rate has been alarming. Of those patients who have been in the study for ten years, 10% have died of a diabetes-related cause (usually heart disease), and 24% have suffered a major diabetic complication. Serious complications are listed in Figure 3.4. At diagnosis 18% had diabetic retinopathy but, 12 years into the study, 53% of patients have diabetic retinal changes.

Patients' experience of the UKPDS

The protocol has been well accepted by patients with NIDDM and it could be used as a model for primary care of diabetes. Because it is a long term research project, the UKPDS has engendered a strong feeling of loyalty among participants, but there is no reason why the same warm atmosphere could not be developed in a practice clinic.

MONITORING AND SELF-MONITORING

4

PATIENTS AS PARTNERS

Self-monitoring allows diabetic patients to be aware of their own glucose levels, to take responsibility for their diabetes and to be as independent as possible. A patient who takes on an active role as partner in controlling his or her diabetes should decrease the amount of time and energy required from a busy doctor and improve the quality of life for both doctor and patient. On the other hand, a patient who remains passive and dependent upon the health care team will take up time and cause frustration on both sides. However, patients will not be able to monitor their own health unless they have been offered a careful programme of assessment and teaching. Individuals with newly diagnosed diabetes will need to understand the implications of the condition. They must also be taught the importance of caution in all aspects of their own health – body weight, foot care and wearing appropriate footwear, prompt treatment of any infections, regular and effective retinal screening and exercise. They need to be aware of the warning signs of hyperglycaemia, ketoacidosis and, most importantly, hypo-glycaemia.

Considering patients as partners follows on from the idea of encouraging adult/adult relationships with health professionals as advisers. It requires us as professionals to delegate responsibility and power.

Motivation is a key factor in partnership in care and this is discussed more fully with special reference to blood glucose monitoring below. The readiness of the individual to begin a self-monitoring programme should be assessed carefully by the health care team and a detailed period of appropriate education provided. Doctors or specialist nurses responsible for starting patients on insulin have to consider how best to address the teaching of self-monitoring of blood glucose levels.

BLOOD GLUCOSE MONITORING

History of urine/blood testing

Some of our longstanding patients recall with distaste the smell of boiling urine that wafted from the hospital diabetic clinic in the late 1940s. Thus the introduction of Clinitest was an aesthetic as well as a revolutionary innovation. For the first time it was simple for patients to monitor their urine in order to assess their metabolic control. Unfortunately, the renal threshold for glucose is 10 mmol/l, which is approximately twice the normal physiological blood level, and this misled people into thinking that negative urine tests indicated that metabolic control was perfect. However, easy urine testing was a dramatic advance and the first step in giving patients control over their own disease.

The first report of patients measuring their own blood glucose levels came in 1976 from pregnant patients in whom scrupulous metabolic control is essential for the wellbeing of the fetus. This was followed a year later by two notable papers in The Lancet, where the domestic use of blood glucose monitoring was described using portable reflectance meters. These were soon replaced by smaller battery-driven meters which

Dr AJC Pickering,
The Village Surgery

Dear Charles
*   I would appreciate your advice about Geoffrey, a gentleman who provides me with one of your "dilemmas". He elects, notwithstanding our advice, to maintain his blood sugar sufficiently high to avoid the risk of hypos, for in the past these have presented suddenly and dramatically as comas. He smokes, and is thus at particular risk of vascular complications. He has background retinopathy.*
*   Geoffrey is a 56 year old married man, recently retired on medical grounds (ostensibly related to his diabetes but, in my view, also related to his wife Barbara's chronic illness and the need to be more active as her carer). Barbara has motor neurone disease which renders her incapable of responding to those acute diabetic emergencies of which they have experience.*
*   Geoffrey argues that, having had diabetes for some 30 years, having a normal blood pressure, no overt signs or symptoms of renal, cardiovascular or vascular disease, and being in his own words "apparently OK", the worst thing he can imagine is another hypoglycaemic coma. My dilemma is that, while I can understand his perspective, I am concerned that he is at risk of MI or proliferative retinopathy in the short term, and other complications in the long term.*
*   His current therapy is soluble insulin/isophane (30/70) mixture twice a day. His HbA1c is about 10%. He refuses to test his blood sugar, not only because he finds it painful (at least he doesn't have neuropathy in his fingers), but because he wouldn't change his habits whatever the blood sugars showed.*
*   I would appreciate your answers to these three questions:*

*   1.   Is there a modification you can suggest to his insulin cocktail which could simultaneously offer better protection against nasty hypos and help to reduce his glycaemia?*
*   2.   Having shared my concerns with him, I feel he now understands the risks he is running and should be supported in his informed decisions. Do you agree?*
*   3.   He has agreed to have regular checks of his optic fundi and I have advised him of the importance of foot care. What other interventions can I suggest that will be effective in his circumstances?*

*   As ever, I would appreciate your views on this matter.*
*   Yours aye,*

Tony

Dr Charles Fox, The Diabetes Centre,
District General Hospital

Dear Tony
      Thank you for your letter about Geoffrey. The problems you highlight
are as follows:
      1.   He keeps his sugars high to avoid hypo, and his HbA1c is 10%.
He is a smoker with background retinopathy and no other complications.
      2.   His wife has motor neurone disease and presumably a poor life
expectancy.
      3.   He refuses to test his blood sugar.
      Everyone with diabetes has to make his own decision and opt for
either good control or fewer hypos. The DCCT has defined the stark
difference in outcome between two groups with different metabolic control.
Good control (mean HbA1c 7.1%) resulted in a very definite reduction in
risk of complications, but a threefold risk of severe hypos. Most people with
diabetes decide subconsciously how much they are prepared to put up with
in the way of hypos. Looking at people's control over time, it is unusual for
the HbA1c to vary, apart from the effect of major life events such as
pregnancy or bereavement.
      As doctors, we are repeatedly reminded of the harrowing
complications of diabetes while most patients usually perceive them as a
black cloud on the horizon. Most people with a chronic disease must cope
with this fear by the belief that "it won't happen" to them.
      I don't know exactly where to place our responsibility as educators. If
the patient is never going to change, there is no point in rubbing his face in
the prospect of blindness and amputation. I suppose that, as doctors/educa-
tors, we tend to protect our own feelings by stressing the positive aspects of
good control. I find it hard to tell patients that they have double the chance
of having a heart attack or a stroke and that there is no evidence that
good control reduces this risk. In practice, it is better to leave this decision
to the patients and ask them, either singly or in a group, whether they want
to hear more about the complications of their disease.
      Barbara's illness must be playing a large part in Geoffrey's present
state of mind. Presumably she will die of her disease in the next few years
and, during the acute stage of grieving, his control is likely to deteriorate
further. Once he is back on an even keel, he will need to re-assess his relationship with his diabetes.
      I have answered your questions in a different order:
      2.   I fully agree that Geoffrey should be allowed to decide for himself
how to resolve the dilemma of better control vs more hypos. The difficulty is
knowing how to give him a balanced picture of the risks he faces. After all,
predicting his actual fate can only be done by gazing into a crystal ball.
Helping him to understand the issues will take several sessions of your time,

with the opportunity for him to express his own ambivalence on the subject.

1. If Geoffrey decides to "turn over a new leaf", his first step must be to start doing blood tests. Since the pattern of his diabetic way of life was laid down before blood testing became routine, he may never have become familiar with the technique. It does cause painful fingers but many motivated people could not imagine life without the information they obtain from frequent testing. As he is on the standard twice-daily insulin regimen, any change would be dependent on the blood glucose results. Apart from alterations in the proportions of the two insulins, the next step would be to have three or four injections per day.

3. Retinopathy may become sight-threatening even after 30 years of diabetes. If Geoffrey decides to tighten up his control after your discussion, there is hard evidence that his retinopathy could enter an accelerated phase for a period of 6-12 months. He needs to attend an annual review for checks on feet, blood pressure and proteinuria.

Yours

made it possible to test blood sugars in the car, the workplace and during leisure activities. There is now available an array of meters which allow blood glucose to be measured accurately in less than one minute, with limited scope for error. These are listed later in the chapter (see Figure 4.3).

Why should patients monitor their own blood glucose?

There is no convincing evidence that self-monitoring of blood glucose (SMBG) improves metabolic control, but it is difficult to see how metabolic control can be improved without measuring the main variable. Most people with diabetes feel guilty that they do not test their blood glucose enough – or indeed ever. Given the results of the DCCT, people with IDDM and an unsatisfactory HbA1c level may want to work to bring it closer to the acceptable range (i.e. less than 7.5%). In simple terms, they have only two options:

■   To increase their daily insulin dose
■   To cut their calorie intake to reduce insulin requirements

People who are overweight may find it worth their while to try the second option though, in practice, it is not easy to decrease food intake permanently – as verified by the slimming industry. Most non-obese people on insulin with a high HbA1c are taking an inadequate dose of insulin because of one or more of the following concerns:

■   They are afraid of hypoglycaemia
■   They actually want to keep their weight down
■   They have never properly been taught the principles of increasing insulin doses in response to raised blood glucose levels
■   They do not want to invest any further time and energy in their diabetes

It important to try to discover the underlying explanation since, if one of the first two concerns applies, there will be resistance from the patient to increasing insulin doses and attempts at improvement will be frustrated. The third explanation is the easiest to correct provided the patient is prepared to believe that "feeling OK" is not the same as good diabetic control. The fourth concern, of course, demands a completely different approach, not forgetting the first recommendation of the British Diabetic Association's response to the DCCT mentioned in the previous chapter: *"The DCCT should not be used as a stick to bully people living with diabetes into meeting clinical targets."*

Figure 4.1

Practical reasons why a person might give up SMBG

	Non-testers (n = 28)	Testers (n = 20)
Lack of time	10	1
Sore fingers	9	2
Testing is messy/bloody	6	0
Inconvenient if at work	3	5
Embarrassing if in public	3	0
Risk of meter being stolen	3	0
Equipment is bulky	1	0
TOTAL	35	8

What determines the success of SMBG?

Not all patients will adhere to self-monitoring regimens. There has been very little research into the reasons why some people carry out self-monitoring of blood glucose while others do not. In Northampton, a recent qualitative study planned and executed by Gill Wade and Anna Fox looked at 48 patients, of whom 20 carried out SMBG (Testers) while the remainder (Non-testers) did not. Interviews identified a variety of reasons why an individual might not continue self-monitoring – these are listed under the broad headings "Practical reasons" and "Emotional reasons" in Figures 4.1 and 4.2. The responses from Testers and Non-testers are presented separately.

The 20 Testers in this study all held in common the view that SMBG was an integral part of living with diabetes. What is not yet clear is how they arrived at this understanding – the answer to this question could affect the way in which SMBG is taught and understood by the professionals. In the meantime, however, we should ensure that any education programme for people with diabetes emphasises, to as great

Figure 4.2

Emotional reasons why a person might stop SMBG

	Non-testers (n = 28)	Testers (n = 20)
No need to test if you feel all right	12	0
Can't be bothered	10	13
Denial of diabetes	9	5
Insulin is essential	6	0
A bad test makes you even more depressed	5	2
No point if you don't use the information	4	2
Will test for someone else, e.g. pregnancy	1	0
Gave up because over reacting to the readings	1	0
Diabetes was controlling my life	1	0
Fear of a high reading	1	2
You give up testing if you're nagged	1	0
Rebellion	1	0
Monitoring is not a high priority	1	0
If you're feeling OK, why inflict pain	1	0
Boredom with continual testing	1	2
Had enough of needles	1	0
Not making the connection between testing and control	0	1

a degree as possible, the connection between monitoring and control. The replies of the Non-testers also have about them an air of hopelessness and futility which highlights the outstanding need for continuing education so that people with diabetes feel motivated to maintain an interest in a difficult ongoing struggle.

How can SMBG be used to improve control?

If a patient is keen to turn over a new leaf, frequent blood testing is the first move in order to find out whether there is a pattern to the raised blood glucose levels. It is crucial that SMBG is done at the four main time points, namely before the three main meals and before going to bed. This need not be done every day, but the timing of tests should be staggered so that a pattern can be established. One is looking at the results to see whether any of the insulin doses can be increased. Patients on the standard mixture of short-acting (soluble) and medium-acting (isophane) insulins twice daily can be given the following advice:

- Aim at blood glucose levels before meals of 4–8 mmol/l
- If blood glucose is high at midday, increase morning short-acting insulin
- If blood glucose is high before the evening meal, increase morning medium acting insulin
- If blood glucose is high before the bedtime snack, increase evening short-acting insulin
- If blood glucose is high in the early morning (i.e. before breakfast) increase evening medium-acting insulin

Patients using pre-mixed insulin, either with pen injector or by syringe, may need to alter the particular 'mix' used for one or both injections.

Figure 4.3 Blood Glucose Monitoring equipment

Meter	Manufacturer	Type of strip	Time	System technology
One Touch II	LifeScan	One Touch test strips	45 secs	No wipe system No timing
One Touch Basic	LifeScan	One Touch test strips	45 secs	No wipe system
Voice Synthesizer	LifeScan	This adapts the One Touch II system for the blind or visually impaired		
Accutrend Alpha	Boehringer Mannheim	BM-Accutest	12 secs	No wipe system Colour chart
Accutrend Mini	Boehringer Mannheim	BM-Accutest	12 secs	No wipe system Limited colour chart
Accutrend	Boehringer Mannheim	BM-Accutest	12 secs	No wipe system Limited colour chart
Reflolux S	Boehringer Mannheim	BM Test 1–44	2 mins	Wipe system Good colour chart
Glucometer GX	Bayer Diagnostics	Glucostix	50 secs	Wipe system Colour chart
Glucometer 4	Bayer Diagnostics	Glucotide test strips	30–40 secs	No wipe system Limited colour chart
ExacTech[1] Companion Pen	MediSense	ExacTech test strips	30 secs	No wipe system
MediSense Card 2	MediSense	G2 Sensor electrodes (test strips)	20 secs	No wipe system
Pen 2	MediSense		20 secs	No wipe system
Hypocount Supreme	Hypoguard	Hypoguard Supreme	60 secs	No wipe system Colour chart
Hypoguard GA	Hypoguard	Hypoguard GA	90 secs	Wipe system Colour chart

[1] Available as 'pen' type or 'credit card' meter

Calibration	Blood glucose range mmol/l	Memory (number of results recalled)	Price	NHS Reimbursement Per 50 strips (Ex/VAT)	Per strip (Ex/VAT)
Programme number for each pot of strips	0–33.3	250 with date & time plus data management facilities	£49	£12.93	26p
Programme number for each pot of strips	0–33.3	Last test result No date and time	£33	£12.93	26p
			£211.20 box alone £250.00 Complete system	– –	– –
Bar code in each vial of strips	1.1–33.3	9, with date	£29	£13.50	27p
Programme number for each pot of strips	1.67–22.2	Last test result	£25	£13.50	27p
Bar code in each vial of strips	1.1–33.3	50 with date and time	£34	£13.50	27p
Bar code in each vial of strips	0.5–27.7	20 with date and time	£29	£14.01	28p
Programme number for each pack of strips	1.4–22.1	10, no date and time	£29	£13.99	£28p
Programme number for each pot of strips	0.6–33.3	10, no date and time	£35	£12.95	£26p
Calibration strip with each pack of strips	2.2–25	Last test result No date and time	£29	£13.45	27p
One step calibration	1.1–33.3	10, no date and time Accessed by Sensorlink	£45	£12.93	26p
One step calibration	1.1–33.3	10, no date and time Accessed by Sensorlink	£45	£12.93	26p
Factory confidence strip	2.2–22.2	14, no date and time	£34.95	£12.73	25p
Factory confidence strip	0–22	10, no date and time	£24.95	£12.21	24p

Splitting the evening dose

It is common for patients on twice daily insulins to have high glucose levels on waking in the morning. Yet if the evening insulin dose is increased the result is a night hypo in the early hours. The explanation for this difficulty is that the medium-acting insulin given before the evening meal has simply worn out before the following morning. The standard solution to this problem is to split the evening dose by having short-acting insulin alone before the meal and delaying giving the medium-acting insulin until bedtime. Patients who have had it drummed into them that insulin must always be followed by food may not find it easy to accept this idea. They should be told that the advice only applies to short-acting insulin and that many people safely give themselves medium-acting insulin at night time.

Conversion to basal/bolus

The basal/bolus regime (three prepandial doses of short-acting insulin and a long-acting insulin dose at bedtime) provides the most flexibility and it should be relatively simple to decide how to adjust the dose in response to the pattern of blood glucose results. In practice, many patients give themselves extra insulin if they discover a high glucose level. This is perfectly logical but can be described as "fire-brigade diabetes" because the insulin is given to extinguish the "fire" of hyperglycaemia. It is more important to take action to prevent the high sugar by increasing the dose of insulin before the appropriate meal the next day.

It has been shown time and time again that the basal/bolus regimen does not, in itself, lead to better metabolic control. The likely explanations are:

■ Inadequate increment in insulin dose for a given increase in food intake – say two extra units before a gargantuan feast

■ Missing the bolus injection completely before a small meal – in particular before a snack lunch

This may be due either to lack of knowledge or to lack of motivation, and it requires some exploration. If the patient is resistant to pre-lunch injections – for whatever reason – there is no point in simply giving expert advice to the effect that the midday injection is as important as all the others.

Blood glucose meters

The chart in Figure 4.3 lists the bewildering range of blood glucose meters now available on the open market. Many of these meters need their own specific strips, which adds to the confusion. Because meters are easily available and relatively inexpensive, many people with NIDDM acquire blood glucose meters which they use inappropriately, often with poor technique. Teaching people how to measure blood glucose must be taken seriously. The newer meters leave less to chance, but there is still no guarantee that without some form of supervision patients are not basing their clinical decisions on false evidence. Patients are often affronted by the suggestion that they may not be using a meter accurately. They may be reassured to know that diabetes nurses and doctors who are using meters regularly are still obliged to take part in a quality assurance programme to verify their technique. It is difficult to keep up to date with all the new meters and a practice nurse will be familiar with one or two different models only. If possible, they should take part in an independent quality assurance programme.

Technique of blood testing

■ Do this carefully and, if teaching other people the technique, keep yourself so familiar with the process that you can do it in your sleep. Restrict the use of the meter to a small number of professionals who test regularly, and

who do not have to read the instructions as they go along.
- Use one of the new finger prickers.
- Provided the finger looks clean and warm, there is no need to wash or sterilise the skin. Make sure the finger is not contaminated with Lucozade or any other glucose-containing material.
- Choose a finger tip where the skin looks thin. Experts often advise patients to use the side of the fingers. However the majority of patients who test their own blood glucose use finger tips. It is easier to form a drop of blood on the tip, and to direct it onto the strip.
- When demonstrating a meter to a patient, remember to discuss maintenance and cleaning of the machine.
- Finger pricking devices are not available on prescription and have to be purchased by the patient at a cost of around £5–8. The lancets can be prescribed on an FP10 and can be re-used many times by the patient.

URINE TESTING

Hospital doctors tend to concentrate on IDDs who are struggling to get their blood glucose levels under control and so urine testing tends to be forgotten. However, urine testing remains the mainstay of monitoring for people with NIDDM, who of course make up the majority of patients with diabetes.

Urine tests rely on the principle that below a certain threshold (about 10 mmol/l), glucose is reabsorbed by the kidneys and urine remains sugar-free. Above the threshold, glucose appears in the urine and can easily be measured.

Which strip should be used?

D*iastix*® (Bayer) or D*iabur*® (Boehringer Mannheim) are the only effective semi-quantitative strips available. Diastix require accurate timing of 30 seconds, which may cause a problem.

Diabur take longer but are not time-critical and should be given to people who do not have a wrist watch with a second hand. Clinistix® should not be given to patients as they are meant for screening for glycosuria and do not give a satis-factory range of results. Some older patients still use Clinitest® which comes with test tube and dropper. It is a bit fiddly but, after a satisfying production of heat and froth, creates a wide range of colours which are easy to distinguish.

How often should urine be tested?

At diagnosis of NIDDM, most patients need to be advised on a sugar-free, weight reducing diet and should be shown how to test their urine. Out of curiosity, most patients test their urine frequently at this stage. In this way they may discover the powerful effect of diet on diabetes, and also find out what tends to "give them sugar" in their urine. If they manage to abolish preprandial glycosuria, they can try testing their urine two hours after a meal. This will provide the most stringent test and patients should not be disappointed if the result is positive. When, and if, a pattern emerges and the results of tests are predictable, it is reasonable to test the urine less often (say one day a week) to check the stability of the control.

Advantages of testing urine *vs* testing blood

- Urine testing is non-invasive
- Urine testing is inexpensive
- There is less room for error

Disadvantages of testing urine vs testing blood

- Urinary glucose is not the important variable
- The threshold for glycosuria may vary with age
- Urine testing is useless in the detection of hypoglycaemia
- Value in IDDM is limited

Dr AJC Pickering,
The Village Surgery

Dear Charles

One of our more remarkable patients is Maureen Groom. Our problem is that whereas her home blood glucose tests are fair (less than 10mmol/l, usually around 7), her HbA1c is consistently around 12%.

She is now 67, developed diabetes over 20 years ago and currently takes Human Mixtard 30 ge twice daily. She is overweight at 108 kg for a height of 1.6 m. She has hypertension controlled (165/80ish) on an ACE inhibitor, and hypothyroidism managed by thyroxine 150 µg daily. Three years ago she had a sub-endocardial myocardial infarction which presented as a sudden improvement in her BP! She has no retinopathy and her renal function as assessed by urine testing and serum creatinine estimation is normal.

We have asked her to do a blood sugar test in our presence and checked her ability to read the colour change on the sticks. Her technique is good and her readings match mine. As far as we can gather, she takes preprandial samples randomly during the week or four times a day one or two days a week. In fact it would appear to be textbook stuff! She is most resistant to the idea of using a meter, claiming she is "too old fashioned to get these machines to work" and we have not pushed the suggestion too far.

I imagine she could be fudging the data in some way, perhaps to "please us" but if this is so, she is in the position of being unable now to admit it. I cannot think of a reasonable form of retreat for her so I suspect we are stuck with this discrepancy. I am tempted to conclude that we can do no more but before doing so would appreciate your comments.

Yours aye,

Tony

**Dr Charles Fox, The Diabetes Centre,
District General Hospital**

Dear Tony

I am afraid the world is full of Maureen Grooms and they are the greatest test of doctors' consultation skills. Certainly, blood sugars in single figures do not square with an HbA1c of 12%. Maureen has brought you the results of her blood tests obtained with a certain degree of discomfort and inconvenience and, basically, you don't believe her data. Quite correctly, you wondered whether technical error was at the root of the problem, but Maureen knows how to measure blood sugar as well as you do. The only explanation is that she is deliberately writing down false results either to deceive you or, possibly, as an act of self-delusion.

There are several different approaches to this difficult situation and GPs, who have highly developed consultation skills, will be familiar with them.

1. Confrontation

This never works as you are openly challenging the trust between yourself and a patient who is probably manipulating the results in order to please you, the powerful "parental" figure.

2. Denial

This is the most tempting approach, whereby you glance at the book of results with mild appreciation and then comment that the HbA1c is still rather high without making any connection between these statements. This approach reinforces the patient's view that you approve of her endeavours while concealment of your negative feelings will avoid placing a barrier between you and your patient.

3. Problem explanation

If there is some time to spare, I try to use this approach. It involves stating the problem from both angles: "Maureen, you have come along with a book of very good results while I also have a raised HbA1c result which tells me that your diabetes is not very well controlled. So we are both faced with a dilemma and, although there are no easy answers, I wonder if you can help us to resolve it". This approach involves being strictly non-judgemental and it is important not to be lured into an admission that you view her results with suspicion. If Maureen accepts that there is a problem, it might even be worth trying the following tack: "Some people bring along to their doctor results which they think will please him, but I would really prefer to know the actual results so that we can work together to get things straightened out".

This last method doesn't always work but it is honest and both parties can end the interview without a bad taste in the mouth.

Yours,

HbA1c (GLYCOSYLATED HAEMOGLOBIN)

When, in 1983, we introduced HbA1c measurements in Northampton, we described to members of the local branch of the BDA that we now had a method of assessing long-term control of diabetes. The patients were not entirely overjoyed at this new development and someone spoke up and described it as "a spy in the cab". It has now become the gold standard for monitoring overall blood glucose levels. The DCCT was based on this measurement.

The clinical and research usefulness of HbA1c derives from HbA1's biochemistry. Glucose is irreversibly bound to haemoglobin (glycosylated) at a rate dependent on the ambient glucose concentration. Haemoglobin is packaged into red blood cells, which have a half-life of approximately 50 days. Brand new red cells that have just emerged from the bone marrow will have a very small proportion of haemoglobin converted to HbA1, while elderly red cells will be weighed down with the stuff. The value is expressed as a percentage which is the average of all red cell HbA1 and therefore reflects the average glucose concentration. Thus HbA1 irons out the peaks and troughs of blood glucose that normally occur in IDDM.

HbA1c is a subgroup of HbA1 which is more specific for glucose and the normal range for HbA1c (4-6%) is therefore lower than that for HbA1 (5-7.5%). A major problem with HbA1c is that there is no universal standard of measurement. There is a variety of methods and each laboratory has its own normal range. This makes it nigh on impossible to compare results from different centres and difficult to compile literature and teaching methods for patients on a national scale.

Figure 4.4   Sample letter about HbAlc result

**The Diabetes Centre,
District General Hospital**

Mrs Mary Brown   Date: 30.9.95
3 Smith Close
Northampton

Dear Mary

I thought you would like to know the result of your
latest HbAlc which tells us what your average blood
glucose level has been over the last two or three months.

The result is *9.4%* (date) *25.5.95*

Anyone taking tablets or diet alone for their control
should be below 7.5%. Here are some guidelines as to
what this result means for people who are taking insulin
to control their diabetes:

Less than 6.5%   Near normal, but results at this level
                  suggest you may be hypo too frequently
6.5%–7.5%   Good control
7.5%–9.5%   Fair
9.5%–11%   Rather poor control
Greater than 11% Blood glucose levels have been
                  worryingly high over the last few weeks

If you would like to discuss changes in your insulin,
please telephone the Diabetes Specialist Nurses on
213000 or 223000

Comments

*It was good to see you in the clinic. This is not perfect but a lot better
than the last result of 11.5%. The hard work is paying off.*

Yours sincerely

Charles Fox
Consultant Physician

Fructosamine

This is a method of estimating total glycosylated protein which has a faster turnover than red blood cells and therefore estimates average blood glucose control over about ten days. However, proteins have a wide range of turnover rates which are influenced by various factors including intercurrent illness. Fructosamine is much cheaper to measure than HbAlc but provides a less accurate representation of metabolic control. Most clinics, therefore, invest in some method of measuring HbAlc.

Practical application

As a general rule patients need an annual HbAlc measurement. There may be a temptation to measure it more frequently but it has been shown that for the vast majority of patients the HbAlc is fairly constant year in, year out. There are of course times when more frequent measurements of HbAlc are justified, in particular in pregnancy, where tight control is all important, and when patients decide to try and improve their control. In these cases an HbAlc can be used to reinforce their success.

Ideally patients should have HbAlc measured before coming to the clinic so the result can be interpreted and discussed. There are now ways of measuring HbAlc in the clinic area but these take up a lot of nurse/technician time and are relatively expensive. If patients have failed to arrange a sample for HbAlc in advance of the clinic, we take blood and let them know the result by post. Figure 4.4 shows a proforma which gives a simple interpretation of the significance of a particular result. It is important to present this in the context of the previous result.

TREATMENT OF INSULIN DEPENDENT DIABETES MELLITUS

5

In the course of an average professional career, a GP will encounter only a handful of new cases of insulin dependent diabetes mellitus (IDDM). When it happens, there might be an instinctive urge to rush the patient off to hospital for the diabetes team to start insulin therapy. This immediate handing over to the hospital gives the patient the message that diabetes is a difficult disease which is beyond the ken of his or her own GP. Perhaps this explains why many patients will consult their family doctor about all sorts of esoteric conditions but insist on asking the clinic professionals a simple query about their diabetes.

How to break the bad news

Because the details of diabetes are not widely known to the general public, anyone disclosing this diagnosis is likely to be met by a barrage of questions. At this early stage, it is worth giving the patient and family a *simple explanation* of the physiology of diabetes and the likely need for insulin. In this way patients first learn about the disease from a doctor they already know and trust. Carry out a *brief examination* looking in

Dr AJC Pickering,
The Village Surgery

Dear Charles,

I would value your advice on how I might avoid making the same mistake twice.

I recently saw Clare, an 18 year old girl with an unusual presentation of diabetes: vague abdominal pains for one week, associated with urinary frequency and non-specific malaise. Her weight had decreased, much to her delight as she had been on a diet (though I cannot imagine why). She had had a nasty sore throat, which she suffered stoically for two weeks, about a fortnight before I saw her with her abdominal pains. She was otherwise well with no past history, personal or family, of note. Her only medication was the combined oral contraceptive, Minulet.

I thought at first she might have a urinary tract problem and was surprised to find neither protein nor evidence of an infection on stick testing the urine. Rather, it contained 2+ of glucose. I then noted the ketones on her breath and having discovered she had vomited that morning, I think my poor solitary cerebral neurone went into panic mode and I arranged her admission. In mitigation, it was Friday night and I was running late.

I am not sure I served this poor kid well. The team on call at the General was very busy, the hospital was bursting at the seams. In the event, she was stabilised on Human Mixtard 30 ge and packed off home within 48 hours with an appointment to see your team four days later and the phone number of the diabetic liaison nurse should she run into trouble in the interim.

Clare and her family thus had one of the most traumatic and ill-supported introductions to diabetes one could imagine. I discovered afterwards that her blood sugar had been 22mol/l on admission and her ketosis was likely due to her not eating all day. I now wish I had taken blood for a blood sugar, packed her off home and gone to see her that evening with the result and the diagnosis so that I might have explored everyone's fears in the comfort and security of her home. I might see about 20 people with diabetes annually but would only expect to see an acute presentation in this age group about once every two years. Surely worth an hour or so of my time? "Good medicine, Bad doctoring" my wise trainer would have muttered if he were very generous; I am more inclined to the "Bad medicine, Bad doctoring" conclusion.

Anyway, the purpose of this letter is to have your advice so that we might refine our practice protocol for the management of diabetes. In partic-ular, would you comment on the following questions:

1. What are the criteria for immediate admission?
2. If we elect to start therapy at home, how much time do we have on diet alone — I presume oral hypoglycaemics are not advisable in the first instance?

3.   How often should we check blood sugars?
4.   Can we safely use a direct-reading glucose meter or do we need the accuracy and reproducibility of laboratory testing?
5.   Should we start with a premixed insulin or a long acting insulin, and should we use a pen injector or ordinary disposable syringes and needles?
6.   Finally, at what point should we involve the liaison nurse?

I feel we have frightened this family unnecessarily and simultaneously reduced the standing and credibility of the community team. I would not wish to repeat this dramatic error!

Yours, mea culpa,

Tony

particular for signs of dehydration, sighing respiration and the unmistakable odour of ketones (pear drops). Check a sample of *urine for ketones* and if positive warn that this indicates the pressing need for insulin by injection. Explain that there is a lot to learn about diabetes in a short time and that the teaching is best done by a specialist nurse who can devote up to an hour a day to the task. Tell patients that you would like to have reports on their progress and that you would be glad to discuss any worries with them or their family. Ideally the process of starting insulin should involve a three way dialogue between hospital, GP and patient/family. A GP who keeps in touch with his or her patient during this difficult time will be given more credit for knowing about diabetes in the future.

Immediately after diagnosis, the overriding anxiety is often a fear of injections. Most people's experience of injections has been venepuncture, which involves threading a large needle into a vein in the antecubital fossa. Some of the fear may be alleviated by letting the patient handle an insulin syringe or

**Dr Charles Fox, The Diabetes Centre,
District General Hospital**

Dear Tony

It was nice to hear your side of the story about Clare, though I think you may have overdone the grovelling. We try to be philosophical about crises on a Friday afternoon. If it's any consolation, we regularly do the same to the nephrologists at the Regional Renal Centre. We have learnt that a weekend is a long time in acute medicine.

I heard about Clare from the SHO who admitted her on Friday. He is experienced in diabetes and didn't just pour into her intravenous fluids and insulin over the weekend and hand her over to me on Monday morning – an equally bad time of the week for most medics. She was feeling pretty sorry for herself and nauseated from the ketones. After two litres of fluid and insulin overnight, she was a new girl and quite positive about the prospect of giving herself injections. She went home on Sunday evening with no abdominal pain and very pleased that you had sent her in. Sue, our new diabetes specialist nurse, has been in touch with Clare and will start the education process after the clinic on Thursday.

I will answer your questions as snappily as possible though I am not so keen on the idea of a protocol for newly diagnosed IDDs. You have pointed out that a newly diagnosed young person with diabetes is a rarity and each case must be judged on its own merits. The main difficulty is to know how "ill" they are using such clues as vomiting, pain, distress, degree of ketonuria and most important the overall impression they give.

1.   Vomiting in the presence of ketones is an absolute indication for intravenous fluids. Other indications include abdominal pain, anorexia, fever, dehydration – and Friday afternoon!

2.   If they are not ill enough to need admission, they should be seen by the Diabetes Team within a few days and it is probably best to leave the insulin to the specialist nurse. It is the "bread and butter" of her job, and she can provide the back up to avoid a disaster. Oral hypoglycaemics don't help much in this situation.

3.   Four blood sugars a day should be enough even at the start of diabetes.

4.   A properly functioning meter used by a properly functioning operator should be accurate enough. Diabetes nurses routinely start patients blood testing early and rely on the results obtained, though of course their technique has to be monitored regularly.

5.   We tend to start with a pre-mixed insulin in young people and a medium-acting preparation in NIDDs who are converting to insulin. I am not sure if this is a scientific arrangement, but it seems to work. We usually introduce new patients to the disposable pen injector but point out that at the moment they have to buy their own needles.

6. I would involve the diabetes nurse early on, to give her as much room for manoeuvre as possible. The diabetes nurse should also liaise between hospital and surgery. In fact Sue will encourage Clare to come and see you in the surgery early next week. Please get back to us if you detect any deep-seated problems.

Yours sincerely (but not smugly)

CHECKLIST

■ **Give a simple explanation of what happens in diabetes to the patient and family**

■ **Carry out a brief physical examination. Do you notice:**
  ● **dehydration**
  ● **sighing respiration**
  ● **odour of ketones?**

■ **Test urine for ketones**

■ **Keep in touch**

pen device. As a rule most newly diagnosed patients remain in a high state of arousal until they have given themselves their first injection with the help of the specialist nurse.

Coming to terms with a chronic illness

People who have worked for a long time as health care professionals forget that they have a different model of disease from patients and their relatives. In the traditional pattern, a patient describes a series of symptoms to a doctor who takes a history, carries out a clinical examination and perhaps arranges a few tests. Having come to a diagnosis, the doctor prescribes some form of treatment (which may be medical or surgical) after which the disease should be cured. Throughout this process, the doctor is active and the patient passive. Patients with no prior knowledge of diabetes will believe that this traditional model can be applied to their own condition. The fact that the patient is asked to do something particularly unpleasant like self-injection reinforces the belief that after a course of injections, the disease will be cured.

Diabetes nurses who work with patients through the early stages of diabetes describe a typical scenario whereby patients react to the initial diagnosis with shock and horror but recover to become almost euphoric as they master self-injection and attain reasonable blood sugars. After three or four months, when things seem to be going well, patients often appear to be indifferent towards their condition. This apathy coincides with the awful realisation that no matter how closely they follow medical advice, this disease will never go away. There follows a grieving process during which the patient mourns the permanent loss of good health.

The only way to turn this round is for the patient to take responsibility for his or her diabetes and to work to incorporate its restrictions into daily life. People with diabetes are barred from some forms of employment (e.g. HGV driving, Armed Forces) but diabetes has been incorporated successfully into most occupations. It is generally believed that patients are more likely to feel confident about their own diabetes if they have been encouraged to make their own decisions from the outset. Professionals should be not be seen as instant problem solvers but as people with experience of diabetes who can work with patients to help them make their own decisions.

Admission to hospital

Historically, newly diagnosed insulin dependent diabetes was an absolute indication for admission to hospital. However with the multiplication of diabetes specialist nurses, most districts have the facility for starting insulin in the community. This difficult task has become a central role of the specialist nurse and there is evidence that patients who start insulin outside a hospital ward are less likely, over the years, to require admission for instability of their diabetes.

COMMANDMENT

**Give intravenous fluids and closely monitor
blood glucose whenever anyone with
diabetes has ketonuria and is vomiting**

This commandment applies as much to the newly diagnosed as to patients already on insulin. It can be difficult to rule out ketoacidosis by simple clinical examination and although we may become blasé about decompensated diabetes, it remains a potentially fatal condition, with a mortality rate of about 5%.

THE IMPORTANCE OF CONTROL

Control, and the different meanings of the term to different people, has been discussed at more length in Chapter 3. To patients, "control" means feeling well in themselves; to the diabetes professionals it is synonymous with a low

HbA1c; and to non-specialists it means the absence of hypos which have been shown in the Diabetes Control and Complications Trial (DCCT) to be a likely consequence of good control. This difference in perception may cause problems with the setting of goals.

The DCCT confirmed that good control rarely happens automatically. It can only be maintained if the person with diabetes incorporates the condition into his or her daily living. This will mean making hour by hour decisions relating to diabetes, frequent monitoring of blood glucose – and the risk of more hypos.

INITIAL TREATMENT

There is a great mystique attached to insulin, and diabetologists have everything to gain by trading on this. Following a standard subcutaneous injection of insulin, the rate of absorption varies enormously. There are many factors which influence the effectiveness and time course of a particular bolus injection:

- Site of injection (arm, abdomen, leg)
- Depth of injection and proximity of blood vessels
- Local blood supply (body temperature, exercise, vasodilatation)
- Current hormonal status (glucagon, epinephrine, cortisol)
- Nutritional state
- Time since last meal
- Rate of gastric emptying

Some of these factors are out of the control of the patient and thus the effect of a given dose of insulin is unpredictable.

Why are doctors wary of insulin?

■ Insulin can only be given by injection and many doctors trained before 1983 were brought up with the confusion of 40 and 80 strength insulins. Happily, since that time, all insulin in UK has been U100 (i.e. 100 International Units per ml).

■ The dose of insulin varies from patient to patient often without rhyme or reason. Patients usually arrive at a dose which seems to suit them, but is not based on scientific principles. However some patients on unconventional regimens have good metabolic control, which increases the impression that the dose of insulin has nothing to do with logic. With the availability of more rational regimens such as basal/bolus (three preprandial doses of short-acting insulin and a long-acting insulin dose at bedtime) and twice-daily fixed-dose mixtures, fewer patients will be on bizarre doses of insulin.

■ The first dose of insulin may cause a hypo, which explains why most specialists start with a low dose and work up.

■ There is a myriad of different insulin preparations and the time actions listed in MIMS add to the confusion. In practice there are only three groups of insulin in production (human, pork or beef) as shown in Figure 5.1.

■ The newly formed Insulin Dependent Diabetes Trust have set out to raise fears about human insulin which may increase the insecurity of GPs. Although there is no scientific evidence to support the theory that human insulin has different properties to animal insulin, many rational patients firmly subscribe to this belief. These people do not like to be told that their own experience is at fault and that science does not support them. Professionals have to take these beliefs at face value and any patients wishing to change the species of their insulin should be allowed to do so freely.

■ The arrival of various pen injectors and different cartridges has increased customer choice but led to some confusion. Consequently, GPs may prescribe insulin of

Figure 5.1 Insulin preparations

1. SHORT ACTING

Vials (human)	Cartridges	Preloaded Pens
Human Actrapid	Human Actrapid Penfill	Actrapid Pen
Human Velosulin Humulin S	Humulin S cartridge	

Vials (animal)
Velosulin Hypurin neutral

2a. INTERMEDIATE ACTING Isophane

Vials (human)	Cartridges	Preloaded Pens
Human Insulatard ge	Human Insulatard Penfill	Human Insulatard Pen
Humulin I	Humulin I cartridge•	

Vials (animal)
Insulatard Hypurin isophane

2b INTERMEDIATE ACTING lente

Vials (human)
Human Monotard
Humulin Lente

Vials (animal
Semitard MC Lentard MC Hypurin lente

3. PRE-MIXED

Vials (human)	Cartridges	Preloaded Pens
Human Mixtard 30 ge	Human Mixtard 30 Penfill	Human Mixtard 30 Pen
	Human Mixtard 10 Penfill	Human Mixtard 10 Pen
	Human Mixtard 20 Penfill	Human Mixtard 20 Pen
	Human Mixtard 40 Penfill	Human Mixtard 40 Pen
	Human Mixtard 50 Penfill	Human Mixtard 50 Pen
Humulin M1	Humulin M1 cartridge	
Humulin M2	Humulin M2 cartridge	
Humulin M3	Humulin M3 cartridge	
Humulin M4	Humulin M4 cartridge	
Humulin M5	Humulin M5 cartridge	

Vials (animal)
Mixtard 30/70 Rapitard MC

4. LONG ACTING

Vials (human)
Human Ultratard Humulin Zn

Vials (animal)
Hypurin Protamine Zinc

the correct type but in the wrong form of pen device. Figure 5.1 should help to clarify exactly what is what.

Types of insulin

1. *Short-acting*

This is standard 'clear' soluble insulin, sometimes known as fast-acting. However it does not really live up to its name. The biological action of soluble insulin can first be detected after 30 minutes, reaches a peak at three and a half to five hours and wears off in eight hours. Insulin analogues with a faster and shorter action are currently undergoing clinical trials.

2a Intermediate-acting *(isophane)*

By adding protamine in equal amounts to soluble insulin, its time action is prolonged with a peak at 4–12 hours and a duration of up to 24 hours. This is the most popular type of intermediate-acting insulin.

2b. Intermediate-acting *(lente)*

Excess zinc is added, delaying its time action to a peak at 7–12 hours and duration up to 24 hours.

3. *Long-acting* (>24 *hours*)

The formation of insulin-zinc hexamer clusters confers a long duration (up to 28 hours) but large inter-patient variation gives a peak varying from 8 to 24 hours. This is declining in popularity.

4. *Pre-mixed* (*mixtures of soluble insulin and isophane*)

This is the most popular type of insulin, the majority being 30/70. There is a full range available from 10/90 to 50/50, but none with a higher proportion of short- to medium-acting insulin. It was shown in 1984 that minor alterations in the proportions of short and medium acting insulin had no measurable effect on blood glucose levels in "real life". However there are strong commercial pressures for manufacturers to produce their present range of finely-tuned mixtures.

Starting insulin

There is no right or wrong way of starting insulin – different specialists have their own favourite regimens. The most important point is to take the patient with you, so that he or she understands what is going on and preferably will come up with his or her own suggestions about dose changes, etc.

We usually start twice daily injections of Human Mixtard 30ge or Human Mixtard 30 Pen. This is the most widely-used mixture and suits beginners. Other people use Human Insulatard ge or Human Insulatard Pen twice daily or go straight onto the basal/bolus regimen. If the patient is unwell with weight loss and heavy ketonuria, we give ten units bd at the outset, but this could be reduced in patients who are picked up early, in whom the blood glucose is only in the low teens.

In general these patients will want to measure their own blood glucose to help with alterations in the insulin dose. In the first few weeks of insulin, the patient will often try very hard to keep all blood glucose levels in the near normal range. They must be warned that this may not be easy, and that they should not be disappointed with occasional sugars in the high teens. In other cases, patients will attain near perfect control with small insulin doses. This honeymoon period, where beta cells recover for a time, really does happen and may last up to six – or even twelve – months. It is a good time for people to adjust to the idea of diabetes, but they must accept that sooner or later they will develop "proper" diabetes.

Adjusting insulin

Most patients are reluctant to take responsibility for changing insulin dose and regard it as the doctor's job. This is a big problem in diabetes, one which must be due in part to the culture which puts dosage of medication into the realm of the professionals, but is also due to our failure to empower patients to take on this task.

The patient must be made aware of the following points:

■ The first step in altering the insulin dose is to measure blood glucose levels. Many patients find this an arduous task which leaves their fingertips sore. However it is difficult to make sensible insulin adjustments without knowing how far the blood glucose level differs from the ideal.

■ When should blood glucose be measured? Ideally the whole day should be spanned by making preprandial measurements and one before going to bed. The tests can be done once or twice a day, staggering the times to get adequate information about each time zone.

■ Look for a pattern to the results – are they consistently high or low at any particular time? If so, the insulin that is working at that time can be adjusted up or down.

■ As a rule, provided the patient feels well, the adjustments need only be small – say two units for each dose, until the respective blood glucose is satisfactory.

■ Always encourage the patient to make the decision about which insulin to change and by how much.

■ Patients who have relatively stable insulin requirements are better off on pre-mixed insulin; this removes the potential error of patients drawing up insulin from two different vials into the same syringe. However, patients who need more short- than long-acting insulin in their mixture will have to mix their own, and a pen injector will no longer be feasible unless they decide to change to the basal/bolus method.

TREATMENT OF NON-INSULIN DEPENDENT DIABETES MELLITUS

6

Diabetes developing in older people has none of the glamour of insulin dependent diabetes, which strikes at children and young people and always needs insulin injections. Many people with non-insulin dependent diabetes mellitus (NIDDM) are unclear in their own minds whether or not they have a serious disease. Patients may describe their condition as "only a bit of sugar" and yet NIDDM carries a two- or threefold increased incidence of cardiovascular disease. Patients diagnosed in their 40s or 50s have a twofold increased total mortality risk. In addition, they also risk all the complications of diabetes, in particular strokes, blindness and amputations. No, NIDDM is not a mild disease.

There are many unanswered questions in the management of NIDDM:

■ Does good metabolic control offer the same protection from complications as the DCCT has demonstrated in IDDM?

■ Does treatment with insulin carry increased benefit over tablet therapy, or could insulin therapy per se increase the risk of cardiovascular disease?

■ What is the optimum treatment for an overweight, poorly controlled patient on a maximum dose of oral therapy?

■ What is the role of acarbose in NIDDM?

■   Does careful control of blood pressure carry any measurable benefit and if so do ACE inhibitors have the edge over other anti-hypertensive agents?

A large multi-centre trial is in progress which attempts to answer these important questions. The United Kingdom Prospective Diabetes Study (UKPDS) was first piloted as long ago as 1979 and the 14 main centres joined in 1982. A blood pressure study was later incorporated into the UKPDS, taking in an additional eight centres. The fact that the UKPDS will need to continue until 1998 demonstrates the difficulty of answering the questions posed above. Until the answers are known, we can only use common sense to help resolve the dilemmas in NIDDM.

DIET

A common reaction of a GP to diagnosing NIDDM is to hand the patient a prescription for glibenclamide. This is quite understandable – the GP may be faced with a patient who is thirsty, tired and (to quote Willy Rushton describing his own diabetes) 'peeing like a mad dog'. The blood sugar may be in the high teens and is clearly not going to respond to diet. So why shouldn't the doctor prescribe a small dose of a familiar drug which will probably make the patient feel a lot better – after all, isn't that what doctors are for? The responses to this question are:

1.   Some patients with blood sugars over 15 mmol/l do respond to diet.
2.   A reasonable period on diet impresses on the patient that this is an essential part of treatment and not just an add-on extra.
3.   During this time when diet is the treatment, patients who are monitoring urine or blood discover for themselves which foods are likely to lead to poor control.

4. This is a time when patients often lose weight and the weight loss is usually reversed after treatment with a sulphonylurea.

COMMANDMENT

Always employ diet as your first line of treatment in NIDDM

COMMANDMENT

Do not use tablets for the first three months

The first of these Commandments is always true but there may be occasional lapses from the second. If, after a month on diet, the patient is still symptomatic with thirst, weakness and fasting plasma glucose greater than 12 mmol/l, further

INITIAL DIETARY ADVICE

■ **Avoid added sugar and sugary food**

■ **Eat normal food at regular meals**

■ **Make cereal, bread or pasta the main part of each meal**

■ **Make meat or cheese a small part of each meal**

dietary manoeuvres are not likely to make any difference. It would then be justified to start a small dose of sulphonylurea, say glibenclamide 2.5 mg or gliclazide 40 mg. Remember that even these small doses may lead to hypoglycaemia.

The patient and spouse need at least one session with a dietitian who has a special interest in diabetes. In households where another family member is responsible for food preparation, it is essential that this person should also be present at this session. A good dietitian will provide:

- A careful diet history
- Specific dos and don'ts
- Imaginative, personalised advice

The main recommendations of the dietitian will be as follows:

1. Work out a food and eating plan which provides an adequate but not excessive amount of food energy.
2. Cut back on fat in the diet to reduce risk of coronary heart disease and arterial disease.
3. As a general rule, avoid added sugar and sugary foods but they can be eaten occasionally. The bulk of the diet should be starchy carbohydrates – fruit, vegetables, beans, wholemeal bread.
4. If overweight, reduce calories by aiming at a high carbohydrate/low fat diet. Agree a realistic target weight.
5. Avoid special "diabetic" foods which are expensive and usually high in calories. Low calorie "diet" foods and drinks may be eaten and drunk.
6. A moderate amount of alcohol is allowable, but take into account its energy contribution. "Low carbohydrate" beer and lagers are usually high in alcohol and calories, and thus not recommended.

TABLETS

Sulphonylureas

All sulphonylureas (Figure 6.1) act by stimulating insulin release from the beta cells of the pancreas. The only difference between one sulphonylurea and another is duration of action. Two of the oldest names in the group have a long half-life, namely chlorpropamide (24–48 hours) and glibenclamide (10–20 hours) and these can lead to hypoglycaemia lasting for days. These are known to have caused several deaths and should be avoided in the elderly and in patients with renal failure.

Apart from hypoglycaemia, sulphonylureas rarely cause side-effects. Very occasionally they cause skin rashes, including erythema multiforme.

Chlorpropamide-alcohol flushing is an idiosyncratic reaction which may be brought about by small amounts of alcohol. It is not usually serious, though may sometimes lead to broncho-constriction. It is relieved simply by changing to a different sulphonylurea.

Gliclazide is a widely used sulphonylurea which seems to be less prone to cause hypoglycaemia. The starting dose is 40 mg bd, increasing if necessary to 160 mg bd.

Weight gain

This is not really a side-effect of sulphonylureas, though many patients will see it as such. Patients starting sulphonylureas have a strong tendency to put on weight, which is largely due to improved glucose control and hence reduction in glucose loss in the urine. This loss may amount to as much as half a pound of sugar in 24 hours, which represents energy that previously could be eaten only to be lost in the urine. Thus improving diabetic control while maintaining the same calorie intake is bound to cause an increase in weight. As the

Dr AJC Pickering,
The Village Surgery

Dear Charles

Ron Bates, a 51 year old father of two, who works as a pharmaceutical representative, presented recently with malaise, weight loss, polyuria and polydipsia. Even I had the wit to test his urine, aided it should be said by his own concern that this might be diabetes, and lo! it was chock full of sugar. His blood sugar was 28 mmol/l. There were no ketones.

As you have doubtless guessed, he was petrified he might be started on insulin and have problems with his employment, though at least he is not an HGV driver. We elected therefore to wait and see what avoiding refined sugars in the diet would do, combined with home monitoring of blood glucose twice daily. After three weeks during which the blood sugar was pretty stable, he returned feeling, if anything, more ill than at the outset. Feeling it was time, and under some pressure (not only from him, for by this stage I was losing my nerve), I started him on glibenclamide (2.5 mg, increasing at weekly intervals by one tablet daily to a maximum of 10 mg twice daily). He began to put on weight and was marginally better in himself and in respect of his blood sugar which fell to 12 mmol/l (fasting sample). However, he is lacking in energy and obviously still not "right".

Ron has met our excellent practice nurse, with whom he discussed the delights of dietary control in the real world – that is he used to grab a coffee in the morning before rushing off to see some GPs 80 miles away, then tear down the motorway munching a sandwich en route to his HQ before rushing back to an evening "drug do" with GPs in the postgraduate centre prior to home at about 11pm. She has prevailed upon him to spread the calories out during the day, focus on unrefined carbohydrates, shun fats and minimise his alcohol intake to legal levels. It was with her that many of his anxieties emerged. There was of course the job, but she was able to counsel him in respect of life's priorities. The prospect of further insurances (he moves around the country quite a lot) was an area she referred back to me. He dropped the bombshell of impotence on her lap, at least metaphorically. This is still the object of some exploration, but she tells me that, curiously, the diagnosis has encouraged real discussions at home with a general improvement in his relationship with his wife, in all domains. Finally she suggested he refer to me about the likelihood of complications.

Thus I find myself in "another fine mess". Ron is not well and I am fairly certain he would feel better on insulin, but should we try metformin plus or minus acarbose first? What is the chance of precipitating retinopathy were we to start insulin? Whereas he will have to let the DVLA know about his diagnosis, is he obliged to tell his firm? I have tried to reassure him that the chances of complications will be much reduced if he can maintain a near normal HbA1C, but then how will he cope with the greater likelihood of hypos?

There is one more fly in the ointment! Ron is very worried that he might have passed on "the tendency" to his daughters, both of whom are married and about to start families. Would you suggest genetic counselling or should we just be very careful to monitor blood glucose (and have a couple of glucose load tests) during pregnancy?

In general my feeling is to avoid stimulating further anxiety while answering his questions and thus not be too proactive, to use that dreadful word so beloved of "management speakers". On the other hand I don't want to allow, by complicity in denial, an avoidable complication – and of course he wants to feel well again! Things were so much simpler in medical school and indeed in the textbooks!

Any advice would be, as ever, most welcome.

Yours aye,

Tony

blood glucose levels fall, patients often experience a sense of wellbeing which may also lead to an increase in appetite.

The UKPDS has shown that patients on sulphonylureas have a significantly greater BMI than their counterparts on diet alone. In the DCCT the group with good control of their diabetes was on average 4.6 kg heavier than the group with conventional control.

Other findings of the UKPDS suggest that of patients with newly diagnosed NIDDM:

- 15% can maintain fasting blood glucose below 6 mmol/l on diet
- 50% on sulphonylureas have fasting blood glucose below 6 mmol/l
- Approximately 15% are not controlled with sulphonylureas from the outset (primary failure), while many patients respond well to sulphonylureas initially but, over time, 30–40% either require the addition of metformin or need to start insulin due to deteriorating beta cell function.

**Dr Charles Fox, The Diabetes Centre,
District General Hospital**

Dear Tony

There is a lot of material in this letter and I am not sure how best to tackle it:

1. Would Ron be better off on insulin?
2. What about his job and lifestyle?
3. How should you address Ron's anxieties about his work, in particular driving, the chances of his family getting diabetes, and the risk of serious complications?
4. What can be done about his impotence?

Insulin

Ron will probably end up on insulin sooner rather than later. However he won't come to any harm in the short term and it is important that when the time comes for insulin, Ron himself agrees that it is the best option. He should certainly try adding metformin – very effective provided Ron can tolerate any side-effects (nausea and diarrhoea). You should agree a plan and set some treatment goals with time limits. For instance he should feel well and have a fasting glucose of less than 8 mmol/l within four weeks.

Acarbose is a logical drug to use in addition to a sulphonylurea. Unfortunately it causes the antisocial side-effect of flatulence which puts off many patients. This unwanted effect moderates with continued use and is reduced by strictly avoiding disaccharides (e.g. sucrose) in the diet.

Lifestyle

Diabetes does not fit well with today's high pressure existence when food is eaten either in a hurry or in extravagant quantities. I find it very difficult to persuade businessmen to make any real changes in their lifestyle. They are usually prepared to make a few minor concessions to diabetes, such as attacking the cheeseboard instead of the Black Forest gateau after consuming a gargantuan main course. The whole problem with diabetes treated with tablets is that it is not really seen as a serious disease until the complications start to bite – or until insulin is needed.

Worries about family and work

Ron is really trying to decide in his own mind whether or not he has a serious disease. He needs to get this off his chest and be told about the genetics of NIDDM. Even if he needs insulin, driving shouldn't be a major problem.

Impotence
        As all cases of impotence, you must first take a
detailed history to discover whether the erectile failure is
absolute. Next examine his foot pulses and look for evidence
of neuropathy. If the impotence is short-lived and if there is nothing to find
on examination, there is a small chance that the problem will improve once
his diabetes is controlled. If Ron remains impotent after a few months of
good control, he could try intracavernosal injections or a vacuum device.
        Yours

At diagnosis it is important to warn patients with NIDDM that after a time of good control using diet or tablets, there may be a progressive deterioration of diabetic control, and that some patients will need insulin.

COMMANDMENT

Remember that all sulphonylureas can cause hypos

Metformin

Metformin enhances glucose uptake into peripheral tissues and reduces output of glucose from the liver. Metformin does not cause hypoglycaemia per se, but may do so in combination with a sulphonylurea. Lactic acidosis is a dangerous complication but is very rare, and mainly occurs in patients with renal, hepatic or cardiac failure. The risk of lactic acidosis is greater when there is tissue anoxia or in the presence of ethanol.

Figure 6.1

List of all sulphonylureas

glibenclamide	Daonil Euglucon }	2.5–15 mg od
chlorpropamide	Diabenese	100–500 mg od
gliclazide	Diamicron	40–320 mg bd
glipizide	Glibenese Minidiab }	2.5–30 mg tds
gliquidone	Glurenorm	45–180 mg tds
tolbutamide	Rastinon	500–1500 mg tds
tolazamide	Tolanase	100–1000 mg tds

In practice the greatest problem with metformin comes from its side-effects which occur in at least 25% of users. These are all related to the GI tract and range from mild nausea to incapacitating diarrhoea. Patients often complain of anorexia together with a metallic taste in their mouth. This explains why of all glucose-lowering agents, metformin is least likely to cause weight increase.

COMMANDMENT

**Always ask about side-effects each time
you see a patient taking metformin**

Side-effects of metformin may develop insidiously over several years and may be intermittent. People therefore need to be re-questioned about side-effects at each visit.

Despite the frequency of side-effects, metformin is a useful and effective agent for lowering blood glucose. In the UKPDS, metformin was used only in patients who were overweight at randomisation, but it proved to be valuable in many cases and has the advantage of not causing hypos. Metformin is a useful adjunct to sulphonylureas and often delays the need for insulin.

Acarbose

This binds to carbohydrate-splitting enzyme receptor sites in the small intestine. Since carbohydrates have to be broken down to monosaccharides before they can be absorbed in the small bowel, acarbose results in less dietary carbohydrate being absorbed. It should be started in very cautious doses (word gets round fast), say 50 mg once a day chewed with the first mouthful of a meal, slowly increasing stepwise to a maximum of 1 g daily in divided doses. Since acarbose is not absorbed from the gut, its side-effects nearly all affect the GI tract. These are similar to the side-effects of metformin with indigestion and diarrhoea. Acarbose also causes flatulence which is exacerbated by the intake of purified disaccharidases such as sucrose. Acarbose on its own cannot lead to hypo-glycaemia but may do so in combination with a sulphonylurea or insulin. Should this occur, it must be treated with glucose since absorption of normal sugar (sucrose) will be slowed by the action of the drug.

WHEN SHOULD YOU CONVERT THE PATIENT FROM TABLETS TO INSULIN?

There is no consensus among diabetologists about when to start NIDDM patients on insulin, although some indications are given in Figure 6.2. The dilemma for the doctor is whether making this change will convert an obese, asymptomatic patient – poorly controlled on tablets – into an even more obese, poorly controlled patient on insulin. It is possible that the soon to be completed UKPDS may yield a clear answer to this problem.

Figure 6.2

Indications for conversion to insulin

---

1. Failure of proper trial on sulphonylurea and metformin
2. Relatively young age (i.e. good control a rational aim)
3. Symptoms (thirst, fatigue, lack of energy)
4. Weight loss, especially if unintentional
5. HbAlc > 10% (very arbitrary)
6. Serious complications reversible by good control, e.g. amyotrophy
7. Pregnancy

NB: Apart from the last, none of these is an absolute indication for starting insulin

The inevitable weight increase after starting insulin is due to:

- Reduced calorie loss in the form of glycosuria
- Increase in appetite as a result of stopping metformin
- An increased sense of wellbeing

In other words the previous relative weight reduction was a pathological state.

Some patients (but not all) feel much better in themselves after starting insulin, with more energy and no need for an afternoon nap. Insulin can be used as a therapeutic trial. If people neither feel better nor have better control after a few months on insulin, they can always opt to go back on tablets.

The patient's attitude towards insulin is all important. Many patients accept that if they manage to lose weight by strict dieting, control will often improve. Patients often prefer a few months grace to get used to the idea of insulin. It is important, therefore, to raise the issue of insulin at an early stage with all "at risk" patients. They will talk to other people about this form of treatment and often receive positive feedback. While patients are deciding about insulin, this is a good time for them to learn self-monitoring of blood glucose (SMBG). Mastering this may help them to reach a decision, so NIDDs who are not already used to SMBG would be well advised to learn the technique.

Some patients return to the clinic with a few pages of high blood sugar values, virtually demanding to start insulin.

MECHANICS OF STARTING INSULIN

Theoretically, NIDDs are suffering from lack of basal insulin. This causes a raised fasting glucose with relatively normal excursions of plasma glucose after meals. Turner and Holman's original solution was to provide a once daily injection of Beef Ultratard, the only true long-acting insulin. Since Human Ultratard has a much shorter duration of action, it is reasonable to use this twice daily, or Human Insulatard, the most widely-used medium-acting insulin. Many UK diabetologists start NIDDs on 30/70 twice daily.

Obesity is a reliable guide to insulin resistance and this will influence the starting dose of insulin (Figure 6.3).

We find that many patients prefer to start straight onto a pen injector which is simpler to use and has a less 'clinical' image than a syringe and bottle. Unfortunately patients still have to purchase their own needles for the pen injectors, but an energetic campaign has been launched by the British Diabetic Association to correct this anomaly. The initial dose of insulin can be increased steadily until preprandial blood sugars are in the range 5–8 mmol/l. In many cases

Figure 6.3

Appropriate starting doses of insulin in relation to body weight

Body weight	Starting dose
<80 kg	10 units bd
80–100 kg	15 units bd
>100 kg	20 units bd

Dr AJC Pickering,
The Village Surgery

Dear Charles

Please can you help me out with the latest gem from my diabetic clinic.

The problem centres on Jasbir Kaur Bhamra, a 65 year old lady who is very overweight (BMI 32) and who on maximal oral hypoglycaemic therapy (glibenclamide and metformin with acarbose) has a fasting blood glucose of 15 mmol/l and an HbA1c of 11%. These values have changed over the last two years no more than her weight. She recently had retinal screening with the non-mydriatic camera and this confirmed the presence of retinopathy that we had noted in the past. She has absent foot pulses and loss of vibration sense but no visible or other neurological disease in the feet. She is hypertensive but her control on an ACE inhibitor is OK at 168/84. Unfortunately she has an ischaemic ECG (undertaken because I wondered whether her "classical" oesophagitis might be anginal). The microalbuminuria present last year has disappeared, thank goodness, with the change in her therapy to ACE inhibitors.

The problem is really me! I am unhappy to let Mrs Bhamra truck along with this poor control for I fear she will develop cardiac complications faster than if we were to switch her to insulin. However I have heard that a change to insulin therapy might exacerbate her weight problem and I am worried that we might precipitate retinopathy. I should say she is quite happy to do whatever I suggest. Actually this is a bit tiresome as I don't feel we are achieving quite the partnership in care that one would like – but that is truly my problem! What would you suggest?

Yours aye

Tony

**Dr Charles Fox, The Diabetes Centre,
District General Hospital**

Dear Tony

You present very clearly the classical dilemma in diabetes. Do you convert a poorly controlled overweight person on tablets into an equally poorly controlled, even more overweight person on insulin?

One of the nice things about the traditional diabetic clinic is that you can quickly trace back the body weight of a patient for as long as they have been attending. When someone who is on the large side tells me that they want to lose weight, looking back through the notes often highlights that the weight has not changed much over the years. Given this unchanging picture, it is rather unrealistic of both doctor and patient to regard significant weight reduction as an option. It is much easier to encourage the patient to accept their present size and to set a target of not allowing the weight to increase.

At the present state of medical knowledge, it just is not known whether tight control of Mrs Bhamra's blood glucose will slow down the rate at which her complications develop. (The DCCT results can only be applied to insulin dependent diabetes.) She is already in quite a lot of trouble with retinopathy and "feet at risk" and in practical terms the best you can do for Mrs Bhamra is to refer her early for laser therapy, control her BP and encourage her to panic if anything happens to her feet. I presume she doesn't smoke.

Since we do not know whether tight metabolic control would improve the outlook with regard to complications, the indications for starting insulin are the same as those in an elderly person with non-insulin dependent diabetes. You need to develop an acute ear for symptoms which can be attributed to hyperglycaemia. Mrs Bhamra may well perceive what the game is and strenuously deny all symptoms ("I've never felt better in my life"). However, tiredness, an unavoidable nap after lunch, thirst, pruritus vulvae and irritability are complaints that can often be corrected by improved blood sugars. If Mrs Bhamra agrees to give insulin a try, you will have to come clean and warn her that as her blood sugars come down, she will lose less sugar (i.e. calories) in the urine and her weight will almost certainly go up.

Yours sincerely

some short-acting insulin will have to be incorporated into the regimen. Thus if blood sugars are acceptable before break-fast and dinner, but high before lunch or bedtime, Human Insulatard ge could be replaced by Human Mixtard 30 Pen.

EXERCISE AND SMOKING

Exercise

Exercise is not high on the agenda in this country of couch potatoes. However it has been shown that regular exercise can reduce the need for sulphonylureas and increase the number of patients who can be controlled on diet alone. In non-diabetic subjects, prolonged exercise leads to a reduction in insulin secretion and an increase in counter-regulatory hormones such as adrenaline and glucagon. In patients on insulin, exercise is a common cause of hypos and these may be delayed for up to 12 hours after exercise due to muscles replenishing their glycogen stores. Most patients take extra food in the form of rapidly absorbed sugars prior to exercise. This means that they have to exercise on a full stomach and of course tend to put on weight. In principle, a more physio-logical way of dealing with exercise is to reduce the insulin dose. Some people with IDDM who achieve high levels of physical fitness for such activities as marathon running find that they can maintain good control with a fraction of their normal insulin dose. However the exact dose needed can only be determined by a process of trial and error with frequent blood glucose monitoring.

Exercise is not a common cause of hypos in patients on diet or tablets, though this is a theoretical possibility for those taking sulphonylureas.

Smoking

Smoking and diabetes are additive risk factors for cardiovas-cular disease and a number of studies have documented this fact. Thus a survey of 120,000 nurses in USA revealed that coronary heart disease was eight times more common in people with diabetes and the risk of fatal and non-fatal heart attacks was even greater in those who smoked. A study of middle-aged Swedish men with diabetes showed that smoking nearly trebled the risk of developing coronary heart disease. It does not appear that diabetes is a deterrent to smoking in young people – in fact they may be more likely to smoke to prove to their peers that they are "normal". Certainly people with diabetes find it no easier to kick the habit than the rest of the smoking population.

All patients who use insulin are at risk of serious disruption to daily life from hypoglycaemia and yet, in the real world, most people come to terms with this hazard. For reasons stated below, it is often a parent or spouse who puts this anxiety into words. For many years, the medical profession has turned a blind eye to the problem of hypoglycaemia and it has only become a popular topic of research within the past ten years.

WHAT IS A HYPO?

It is useful to think of hypoglycaemia as having two separate effects:

1. **Adrenergic effects**

   These result from counter-regulatory processes in response to this physiological catastrophe. In particular, adrenaline and glucagon cause a rapid release of glucose from the liver and patients rely for warning on the "fight and flight" symptoms of sweating, tremor and palpitations. In practice, most patients work out their own warning symptoms which do not necessarily coincide with textbook descriptions.

2.   **Neuroglycopenic effects**
The brain has high energy requirements and relies almost entirely on glucose as a source of fuel. Cerebral function is measurably impaired when plasma glucose falls below 3.5 mmol/l, and at lower levels behaviour becomes irrational and the patient often denies the possibility of hypoglycaemia with great vigour. If untreated, there follows paralysis, hemiplegia and, eventually, coma.

Definition of hypoglycaemia

There is a problem with definition. In medical terms hypo-glycaemia consists of a plasma glucose concentration less than 3.5 mmol/l at which point counter-regulatory processes come into play to try and correct the problem. From the patient's point of view a "hypo" is a subjective experience resulting from a low blood glucose. A mild hypo causes such symptoms as sweating, tremor, palpitations or a feeling of panic which the patient can correct by taking some form of sugar. A hypo is more severe if it interferes with normal activity and other people are involved. Family, workmates or schoolfriends may assist in providing sugar. A hypo is serious in patient's eyes if there is loss of control culminating in coma. In practice, the patient's classification on functional grounds is more useful than a scientific measurement of the blood glucose. Glucose meters are not particularly accurate at the low end of the range and of course one must question the ability of anyone in a state of neuroglycopenia to measure their own blood glucose with accuracy.

Fear of hypos

Most people starting insulin are curious rather than terrified about hypos. They almost look forward to having their first brush with hypoglycaemia. Once they have experienced the condition, however, most patients are wary – although it is rare in the detached atmosphere of a medical consulting room for a patient to express anxiety about hypos. At a National Youth Diabetes Conference, where replies were anonymous, 22% of participants admitted that they were "terrified" of hypoglycaemia. However people on insulin who also hold a driving licence may be reluctant to describe disturbing incidents to the doctor responsible for certifying their capacity to drive. In addition neuroglycopenia reduces awareness and blurs memory of a significant hypo.

Night hypos

A spouse or parent will usually describe more accurately the impact of hypoglycaemia, often with strong feelings of frustration and anger. Night hypos are particularly disruptive and may keep the carer up for several hours dealing with someone who is obstreperous and confused. The patient, however, is likely to wake up the following morning as if from a good night's sleep.

Carrying sugar

It is puzzling how few young people with diabetes actually carry around with them some form of sugar – Dextrose tablets or a chocolate bar. The reason they give for not taking this simple well-known advice is that they would only eat their supplies of sugar on impulse when their blood sugar level was not actually low. Many young drivers on insulin admit that for the same reason they don't carry sugar in their glove compartment and that if they feel they are hypo while at the wheel of their car, they drive 'to the next petrol station' to buy something suitable from the shop. Without doubt many drivers with diabetes do follow the advice to carry sugar and treat symptoms of hypoglycaemia immediately, but we must understand that in practice some patients do not take these simple precautions to reduce the risk.

WARNING OF HYPOS

This is always a difficult topic to discuss with patients. A few patients admit to losing completely their warning symptoms of hypoglycaemia but the majority retain some alarm signal that their blood glucose is low (Figure 7.1). However, it can be shown experimentally that there is a measurable loss of cognitive function at a level of blood glucose higher than that which causes symptoms. So patients are in the difficult position where they may already be slightly irrational with impaired judgement before they themselves can be aware that all is not well. This is not an easy concept to get across to patients who understandably believe that if they feel all right, then they are all right.

Figure 7.1

Signs and symptoms of hypoglycaemia

Hypoglycaemia is LOW blood sugar. Also called a hypo, a reaction or an insulin reaction

It has a FAST onset

- Tingling of the lips and tongue
- Weakness
- Tiredness
- Sleepiness
- Trembling
- Hunger
- Blurred vision
- Palpitation
- Nausea
- Headache
- Sweating
- Mental confusion
- Stumbling
- Pallor
- Slurred speech
- Bad temper
- Change in behaviour
- Lack of concentration
- Unconsciousness (hypoglycaemic or insulin coma)

How common are hypos?

The epidemiology of hypos reveals some worrying findings:

- People with diabetes under-report hypos
- 10% of people on insulin have had a severe hypo in the previous year

In the "tight" control group of the DCCT, patients on average had a severe hypo every 20 months. The severe hypo rate was reduced to one in five years in the groups with less tight control and the hypo rate fell in both groups as the study progressed.

Causes of loss of hypo warning

These can be listed, briefly, as follows:

1. Neuropathy
2. Duration of diabetes
3. Tight control (loss of symptoms can be reversed by running higher blood glucose levels)
4. Possibly, human insulin

Neuropathy

Many of the symptoms of hypoglycaemia (sweating, tremor, palpitations) are mediated by the autonomic nervous system. Autonomic neuropathy may be one of the most debilitating complications of diabetes and, in particular, patients with severe autonomic damage may be devoid of hypoglycaemic warning systems and, consequently, have to run high sugar levels to reduce the risk of hypo.

Duration of diabetes

Most patients after a decade or so of diabetes announce that their warning of hypos has become more subtle and they have to be more attuned to the rather feeble messages.

Tight control

Diabetes is an unjust disease and it has been shown that people who achieve tight control of their blood sugars do not have warning symptoms until the plasma glucose levels are lower and, therefore, there is less leeway before they become neuroglycopenic and often irrational. Since we now know from the DCCT that people with tight control are more likely to have serious hypos, it is really a double insult that they also have less warning.

Human insulin

A number of patients feel very strongly that changing from animal to human insulin is responsible for their own loss of warning of hypos. There have been many attempts to find a scientific basis for this observation, but to no avail. However, this does not shake the conviction of such patients and their outrage has fuelled the development of the Insulin Dependent Diabetes Trust. Most patients will have heard of this phenomenon through the grapevine. If a patient is showing signs of unhappiness over problems with hypos, it is always worth offering a change to the porcine equivalent of the insulin being used.

Minimising the risk

There are also good reasons why people on insulin may minimise the true risks of hypos. Such underestimation may be a coping mechanism to reduce their own levels of anxiety. People may not wish to think too hard about the risk because of fears of losing their driving licence. In addition, neuroglycopenia may reduce the person's awareness of hypoglycaemic episodes.

TREATMENT OF SEVERE HYPOS

A severe hypo is one where the patient needs help from a third party. This may simply be help with opening a bottle of Lucozade or finding the Dextrose tablets. It is standard for a patient to manifest signs of neuroglycopenia by truculent or even violent behaviour, with a firm denial that anything is amiss. A close relative who is familiar with the hypo experience will overrule the patient and try to cajole him or her to accept some form of glucose. On the other hand, a workmate who is seeing a hypo for the first time may be deterred by these protestations and leave the patient to sink or swim. If untreated, the patient is likely to become floppy and unable to stand. He or she may complain of blindness or show obvious signs of hemiplegia. The next stage is coma often accompanied by convulsions. Parents need to be warned about this possibility which always comes as the most unpleasant shock.

If you arrive during the process of a hypo, the first priority is to try and make a firm diagnosis. A reliable spouse or parent may provide enough evidence but, in most cases, it is reassuring for the nurse or doctor to measure a finger prick glucose. This in itself may be a challenge in a restless, irritable patient and it is important to ensure that the finger tip is not contaminated with any form of glucose. This has been recorded as a potentially dangerous artefact while measuring capillary blood glucose in a casualty department.

Having confirmed that the glucose is less than 4 mmol/l, try to persuade the patient to take some form of glucose. Dextrose tablets are easy to carry about but, if the hypoglycaemic patient is confused and drowsy, the tablets may remain in the mouth being solemnly chewed and never actually reach the stomach. For this reason, a sugary fluid may be more effective.

After a prolonged severe hypo, it is normal for the patient to remain confused or weak for a time, even though the plasma glucose has returned to normal. This is akin to the post-ictal state following an epileptic convulsion.

Amount of glucose needed

Most textbooks and manuals suggest that a hypo can be corrected by taking three or four glucose tablets, each consisting of 3 g of glucose. This is often a huge underestimate. It is not unusual for patients to take a whole packetful of tablets (47 g). Young adults who wake in the night to find themselves hypo may stumble down to the kitchen where they devour prodigious quantities of food. One lad described eating three bowls of Weetabix followed by a whole Swiss roll. Many people who are truly hypo have a strong compulsion to gorge, presumably as a defence mechanism.

Hypostop

This can be prescribed on an FP10 and is presented as an opaque, gluey gel in a plastic bottle. The gel has an inoffensive flavour and the whole bottle contains 30 g of glucose. About half the contents can be squeezed into the side of the cheek where it will dissolve to be swallowed.

Glucagon

Glucagon can be given either subcutaneously or intravenously and causes the release of glucose from the liver, thereby correcting severe hypoglycaemia. Glucagon is prescribed in a

Figure 7.2

Essential patient information on insulin and hypoglycaemia

What every person on insulin must know about diabetes	What other people must know about diabetes
■ NEVER stop insulin if you feel ill or sick. Check your blood sugar – you may need extra insulin even if you are not eating very much	■ NEVER stop insulin in case of sickness (no apologies for repeating this)
■ If you are being sick, try to keep up a good fluid intake (at least 2½ litres (4 pints) a day). If you are vomiting and unable to keep down fluids, you probably need to go to hospital for an intravenous drip.	■ Repeated vomiting, drowsiness and laboured breathing are bad signs in someone with diabetes. They suggest impending coma and can be treated ONLY in hospital
■ ALWAYS CARRY SUGAR or some similar quick-acting carbohydrate on your person	■ A person who is hypo may not be in full command of his or her senses and may take a lot of persuasion to have some sugar. Jam or a sugary drink (e.g. Lucozade) may be easier to get down than Dextrose tablets. Hypostop, a glucose gel, may be useful
■ NEVER risk driving if your blood sugar could be low. People with diabetes DO lose their driving licences if found at the wheel when hypo	■ NEVER let someone drive if you suspect they are hypo. It could be fatal
■ REMEMBER physical exercise and alcohol are both likely to bring on a hypo	

GLUCAGON RULES

■ Give glucagon earlier rather than later, as soon as the patient is too uncooperative or conscious to tolerate Hypostop

■ Show the patient and carer how to use glucagon using a pack which has outlived its shelf-life

■ The full dose of I mg is pharmacological rather than physiological. Give half the dose (even less in a child), and wait five minutes to see whether it has been effective. If not, give the remainder

pack containing a bottle of powder and a syringe containing diluent. Preparing the solution can be a complex task for a lay person, particularly one in a state of panic.

Glucagon may take between five and 15 minutes to take effect, and it is is always said that on regaining consciousness the patient should be given sugar by mouth to maintain blood glucose at a normal level. However, people often suffer a headache and feel nauseated after a bad hypo – so the last thing they want is a glass of Lucozade or a slice of bread and honey. Provided there is not thought to be a large bolus of insulin remaining at the injection site, it is safe to allow the patient to wait for the next meal before eating. After recovering from a night hypo, the patient can be allowed to go back to sleep.

SULPHONYLUREAS AND HYPOGLYCAEMIA

It is one of the best kept secrets in medicine that all sulphonylureas can cause hypoglycaemia. The onset is often more insidious than with an insulin hypo and, characteristically, presents as confusion or mimics a stroke. Because of the patient's age and classical presentation, the true diagnosis is often missed. Thus many fatal cases of hypoglycaemia have been reported in older people taking sulphonylureas. Insulin hypos do not usually recur once corrected, and patients coming to casualty can be allowed home once they are normoglycaemic and compos mentis. However, a hypo due to a long-acting sulphonylurea such as glibenclamide or chlorpropamide may last for more than 24 hours. Such patients should always be admitted for observation and given intravenous glucose.

OTHER HYPOGLYCAEMIC AGENTS AND HYPOGLYCAEMIA

Metformin

Metformin does not act by increasing pancreatic insulin secretion, and therefore cannot cause hypoglycaemia on its own. Of course, adding metformin to any sulphonylurea may bring the glucose down below normal and lead to problems. If this happens, the dose of either drug could be reduced to keep blood glucose in the normal range.

Acarbose

Likewise, acarbose can cause hypoglycaemia only in combination with a sulphonylurea. Because acarbose delays absorption of all polysaccharides, any disaccharide (e.g. sucrose) or starch will not correct hypoglycaemia effectively. Patients taking acarbose need to be warned to take glucose (Dextrose tablets, Lucozade or Hypostop) if they become hypo.

DIABETES AND PREGNANCY

8

The problems and disasters of diabetic pregnancy may make gloomy reading, but for diabetic specialists the care of a pregnant woman can be the most joyful part of their work. Doctors and nurses must work closely with diabetic mothers and can take pleasure in the efforts of patients who work hard to achieve excellent control of their diabetes. Care should be based in a specialist unit with diabetologist and obstetrician working together, an arrangement which significantly reduces perinatal mortality. However, the GP must share some of the care, to provide a point of contact in the community, and emotional support when the going gets tough – as it often does during a diabetic pregnancy.

With so much at stake, it is easy for professionals to make impossible demands on their patients. How, for example, can a mother with morning sickness hope to keep preprandial glucose values between 3 and 5 mmol/l, and not exceeding 7 mmol/l after meals? Of all branches of diabetes, this is one where doctors and nurses may readily take leave of the real world, inhabiting a different planet from their patients.

Dr AJC Pickering,
The Village Surgery

Dear Charles

I would be grateful if you might agree to see Suzanne Jones soon in the joint obstetric/diabetic clinic.

Suzanne is a 28 year old accounts clerk for a large local company who is delighted to find herself pregnant after a stormy past obstetric history. She developed diabetes when she was 14 and has had a difficult time in this regard too. She is married to a manager in a food store.

She stopped taking the contraceptive pill when she has 22 in order to start a family but was frustrated by difficulty in conceiving for two years. Sadly, when she did become pregnant, the implantation was ectopic, resulting in a salpingectomy at eight weeks. In her next pregnancy, two years later, Suzanne had a miscarriage at five weeks. She is now seven weeks into her third pregnancy.

There have been no obvious obstetric problems so far though I am sure Suzanne should have an urgent ultrasound scan to confirm an intrauterine pregnancy and her dates since her cycle is rather erratic.

A major problem is her diabetes. From the time of her diagnosis she has relied on insulin, latterly Human Mixtard 30 ge, but has not been able to manage her diabetes very well, commonly running an HbA1c of 11%. Her maternal grandmother was a NIDDM and died young after a series of tragedies — blind at 42 she developed severe ischaemic heart disease in her late 40s, underwent a series of amputations in her early fifties and then died of renal failure at 58. You will not be surprised to learn then that Suzanne is somewhat fatalistic and has consistently, in effect, denied her own condition, avoiding most of the monitoring she was offered, preferring to run a high blood sugar than suffer hypos. She has for many years been a bit overweight, BMI 29, and monitors her blood sugar only if she feels she might be getting a bit low.

Since Suzanne joined our list, we have tried to act as advisers in what has been a damage limitation exercise. Paradoxically, she was desperate to have a family, seemed to understand the relationship between diabetic control and successful obstetric outcome, but failed to "toe the line". I have not managed to find the right approach with her.

In other respects, she is both healthy and careful. She has had no other major medical episodes, consults us only rarely and then appropriately, does not smoke and drinks alcohol only occasionally. I sometimes wonder if she avoids the profession and thereby, as she sees it, her "fate".

I should add that she had a miserable and most damaging encounter with a doctor during her first pregnancy — it seems he berated her for her apparent insouicience and told her that she "should grow up". I have no information other than her reports and a bland letter about this consultation, but I have no reason to doubt her.

I imagine, and I have told Suzanne, that her best chances of a successful outcome to her pregnancy require that her care should be primarily directed by you though I would be pleased to chip in as required. She is scheduled to meet our midwife and our health visitor in the next few weeks.

Yours sincerely

Tony

PATHOPHYSIOLOGY

Why is diabetes a problem in pregnancy?

Before we consider the clinical aspects of diabetes in pregnancy, it is important to understand the physiological principles which underlie the problems of diabetic pregancy. As in many other diabetic scenarios it appears that glucose is the main culprit, causing the host of difficulties that haunt what should be a happy event.

Clinical and experimental studies support a hypothesis that high concentrations of blood glucose cross the placenta from mother to fetus, which responds by increasing output of insulin from the beta cells (Figure 8.1). This, in turn, promotes the deposition and storage of protein, glycogen and fat. As well as the beta cells, liver, spleen, heart, adipose tissue and adrenals are enlarged and there is evidence of increased blood production. The hypothesis now incorporates the effects of other substances, including amino acids, which stimulate insulin production. The objective of treatment in diabetic pregnancy is to keep the mother's blood glucose levels as close to normal as possible. Centres which provide well-organised expert antenatal care, and which pursue tight control of the diabetes, have seen in a fall in perinatal mortality from 30% in the early 1950s to a current rate of 1%.

**Dr Charles Fox, The Diabetes Centre,
District General Hospital**

Dear Tony

The world of diabetic pregnancy is often poignant and Suzanne's story is a good example. This is a "precious baby" in someone with only one tube remaining, who has difficulty conceiving and has already lost two babies.

It is interesting to hear about her Granny as a diabetic role model. People with first hand experience of diabetic disasters either seem to have perfect control or the sort of fatalism that you describe so well in Suzanne.

In practical terms, we must see her soon and arrange a dating scan before 10 weeks. The HbA1c of 11% is a worry and certainly exposes her baby to increased risk of congenital abnormalities. I am never sure how to discuss this after organogenesis has taken place. Every pregnant woman has a dread of giving birth to a deformed baby and if the disaster is in some way of her own making, the feeling of guilt must be overwhelming. One approach is to stress the importance of the anomaly scan at 20 weeks so that the mother is at least aware of the possibility of abnormality. However, it is not the job of the medical profession to induce guilt over a state of affairs which already causes huge unhappiness. I don't think there is a "right approach" to Suzanne, but we must try to provide support and stay "with her" rather than add to her bad feelings.

There certainly is a wrong approach which our colleague illustrated but I must not be too pious about this dreadful behaviour. These cases always engender strong feelings, partly because we know that if things go wrong it falls to us to pick up the pieces. It is all too easy to offload our own fears and anxieties onto the patient or her partner. We can see "the party line" so clearly and for every Suzanne, there are many women who do stick to the straight and narrow. At the end of the day she has to make her own decisions and we must do our best to work with her.

Yours sincerely

Figure 8.1 Effect on the fetus of insulin deficiency in the mother

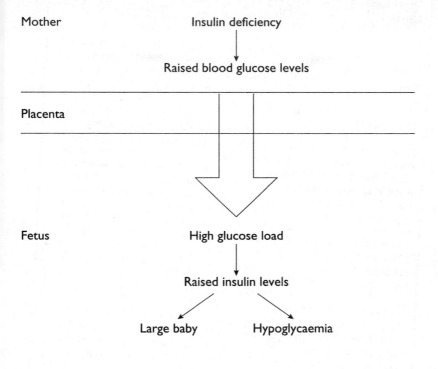

COMMANDMENT

Advise your patient to plan the pregnancy

Diabetes commonly presents during pregnancy because the process of gestation in the non-diabetic woman makes considerable demands on the insulin-producing cells. This is largely due to human placental lactogen (HPL), a hormone with an anti-insulin action which originates in the placenta. As pregnancy progresses, the pancreas has to double its insulin output in order to keep blood glucose levels normal.

WHAT CAN GO WRONG IN DIABETIC PREGNANCY?

By convention, a distinction is made between those problems which affect the baby and those which affect the mother. This may seem a pointless distinction in a union as close as that between mother and fetus. Even when the baby is the main casualty, the mother is profoundly affected. However, it helps to consider who is at greatest risk from each problem.

Risks to the baby

Congenital abnormality

Severe congenital abnormality affects about one baby in 100. In diabetes this risk is increased three- to fourfold, and is directly related to blood glucose levels in the first trimester. If blood glucose levels are kept near normal during fetal development, the extra risk is virtually abolished. In mothers with poor control in the first trimester, the risk may be as high as 10–20%. Since fetal damage may occur before the mother knows that she is pregnant, pre-conception counselling is of paramount importance.

COMMANDMENT

Aim to keep blood glucose levels as near normal as possible, e.g. 4–6 mmol/l before meals

Spontaneous abortion

When poor diabetic control causes major fetal or placental abnormalities, first trimester miscarriage is likely.

Large babies

Babies of diabetic mothers are often overweight with a bloated plethoric appearance, described as macrosomia. In consequence, the caesarean section rate is much higher in diabetic mothers. If blood glucose levels run high during the final weeks of gestation, the baby may increase in weight dramatically. Big babies deliberately delivered early are not small for dates, but they are premature, and the risks of prematurity must be balanced against allowing term delivery of an unhealthy macrosomic baby.

Prematurity – respiratory distress syndrome

Before tight control was routine during pregnancy, planned early delivery was the norm, sometimes as early as 32 weeks gestation. The obstetrician and diabetologist's problem was then transferred to the paediatrician, and a stormy course for the baby in a Special Care Baby Unit was the likely outcome. When control is poor, or pre-eclampsia occurs, decisions about the timing of delivery are still difficult.

Small babies

Some babies born to diabetic mothers are actually small for dates. This paradoxical phenomenon usually occurs in mothers with advanced diabetic complications and generalised atheroma. Placental blood supply is poor, fetal nutrition suffers and the baby is underweight.

Maternal ketoacidosis

Diabetic ketoacidosis is dangerous. The mother's mortality risk is 5%. In pregnancy, the fetal mortality rate is around 50%.

Hypoglycaemia

Maternal hypoglycaemia does not harm the fetus. However, after delivery, the baby is unable to scale down insulin release and becomes hypoglycaemic when suddenly deprived at delivery of (maternally derived) high glucose intake. Once identified, the problem can be controlled with glucose feeds. Within a matter of days, the baby's beta cells settle down and produce appropriate amounts of insulin.

Intrauterine death

Whilst this may occur unexpectedly towards the end of a normal pregnancy, it is more common in diabetic mothers. Obstetricians are usually reluctant to allow gestation to advance beyond 39 weeks and certainly want to induce delivery at term.

Risks to the mother

Unstable diabetes

This is a particular problem early in pregnancy when morning sickness strikes. It must be frightening for a mother to have her morning dose of insulin only to become utterly nauseated at the thought of breakfast. Food intake and insulin dose need to be flexible, while maintaining good control is of overriding importance.

Pre-eclampsia

Diabetic pregnancy carries double the normal risk of pre-eclampsia. Progression to fulminating toxaemia may be lethal. In the common (milder) form, it threatens the fetus by reducing placental function. The decision about when to intervene and deliver the baby may be difficult.

Hydramnios

This is also more common in diabetes. It is uncomfortable, but does not present a serious risk to the mother. It is associated with fetal abnormality and can lead to premature labour and cord prolapse.

Hypoglycaemia

Women with diabetes are encouraged to maintain superlative control throughout their pregnancy. As demonstrated by the DCCT, this increases the risk of severe hypoglycaemia. Whilst maternal hypos do not harm the fetus in any way, they disrupt the mother's life. Patients require clear warnings about possible problems from hypos (e.g. in driving), and partners must have a supply of glucagon and knowledge of how to use it.

Caesarean section

In most centres the section rate is 10–15% in non-diabetics. However, it is 50% in diabetic women.

Retinopathy

Many diabetic women who become pregnant will already have some degree of retinopathy. This is not usually a matter for concern but, in about 20% of women, retinopathy will fulminate and require repeated laser treatment through pregnancy and beyond. It is well known that improved diabetic control may provoke a striking but transient deterioration in retinopathy which is the likely explanation for this phenomenon during pregnancy.

Nephropathy

Patients with persistent proteinuria, indicative of nephropathy, are likely to have a more stormy course during their pregnancy. As pregnancy progresses, the degree of proteinuria tends to increase and may cause oedema. Hypertension and placental insufficiency are also common problems. However, there is no evidence that pregnancy irreversibly accelerates the progression of diabetic renal disease.

CLINICAL PRESENTATIONS OF DIABETES AND PREGNANCY

Division into three clinical categories is useful:

1. Women with diabetes who have planned the pregnancy and have deliberately achieved good metabolic control before conception.
2. Women whose diabetes is not well controlled. Members of this group may present late to the antenatal clinic.
3. Women whose diabetes comes to light during pregnancy. The majority of these are detected by screening "at risk" women (see Figure 8.2). However, some women with IDDM simply happen to present while they are pregnant. They have usually lost weight and are ketotic. They need to start insulin immediately.

Dr AJC Pickering,
The Village Surgery

Dear Charles

I'd appreciate your advice regarding glycosuria in pregnancy as we would like to develop a practice policy in order that we might have a coherent (and appropriate) strategy.

The current position is that we test the urine of all pregnant patients when they attend. We should have available the family history in respect of diabetes and the previous obstetric history regarding birth weights and glycosuria.

We can't quite decide on which of the following is safe and expeditious:

1. Glycosuria should be followed by a 50 g glucose load test (GLT), that is a blood sample one hour after 50 g glucose taken by mouth. This is our current practice but we are concerned that we may miss some patients with abnormal glucose tolerance, for example if they happen to provide a urine sample after an overnight fast.

2. Glycosuria in the absense of any other features (family history, past history, large for dates) should be followed by a fasting blood glucose (FBG) which if abnormal should be followed by a GLT. The issue here is that the GLT is unpleasant and logistically moderately tricky; is a FBG any better than a urine test in this context?

Glycosuria associated with any sinister history or features should be followed by a GLT.

3. All women regardless of history or urine findings should have a fasting blood glucose in the first and third trimesters followed by GLT as indicated. I know, however, that fasting blood tests are not well regarded by patients who may be feeling nauseated.

4. All women should have a GLT in the first trimester and then further GLTs as indicated by urine tests. This is unusual in UK practice and it is a bit of a pain for the patients but it should indicate all those at risk of gestational diabetes.

There is then the whole business of how to manage abnormal glucose tolerance in pregnancy. We are presuming that the GLT is as good as a formal glucose tolerance test for the purposes of diagnosis; certainly it is easier and cheaper. Once abnormal tolerance is suggested our practice is to refer to the joint diabetes/obstetric clinic; is there anything else we could do?

Would you kindly let us have your views on this matter and, in passing, tell me what proportion of women with abnormal tolerance develop gestational diabetes, and what proportion of these develop diabetes proper? Would this last group tend to IDDM or NIDDM and do we know why?

Yours sincerely

Tony

**Dr Charles Fox, The Diabetes Centre,
District General Hospital**

Dear Tony

You were very astute to present a number of different options for managing suspected diabetes in pregnancy. A research worker recently looked at the protocols for managing diabetes and impaired glucose tolerance in pregnancy in 17 hospitals in the same region. There was a huge variation in the criteria for diagnosing diabetes in different centres so that a particular blood glucose level would result in insulin therapy in one hospital while, in the neighbouring clinic, an identical patient would be sent on her way with some dietary advice if she was lucky.

I will comment on each of your suggestions:

1.   The glucose load test (GLT) was developed as a useful screening test which can be carried out on the spot. The patient does not need to be fasting and one hour after taking 50 g of glucose drink, a plasma glucose is measured. Since a lot may depend on the result, the measurement should be made in the laboratory rather than using the surgery blood glucose meter. If the one hour sample is less than 7.5 mmol/l, the patient can be reassured that all is well. If it exceeds this threshold, a formal oral glucose tolerance test should be carried out.

2.   Instead of a GLT, glycosuria prompts only a fasting blood glucose. This is not an adequate screening test for diabetes in pregnancy where fasting levels may often remain normal while the post-prandial result may be alarmingly high. Pregnant women often object to drinking a concentrated glucose solution. However, the 50 g test is not particularly arduous and it does not have to be drunk on an empty stomach.

3.   All women should have a fasting glucose measurement. This is not such a crazy idea as the prevalence of gestational diabetes is quite high and not all patients have one of the recognised risk factors for this condition. For the reason above, however, a fasting glucose measurement is not enough and some form of tolerance test would have to be carried out.

4.   Universal GLT in the first trimester is a logical approach to the problem and would theoretically pick up every case of gestational diabetes and impaired glucose tolerance. Against this would have to be set the unnecessary anxiety caused to the large number of women with a raised GLT who then went on to have a normal 75 g GTT.

5.   You did not mention this, but HbA1c has been suggested as a screening test. Unfortunately, it is not sensitive enough. There is also the difficulty that during pregnancy there is an additional production of "young" red blood cells, thus reducing the mean HbA1c result.

Having diagnosed abnormal glucose tolerance in pregnancy, it is worth a referral to the joint diabetic antenatal clinic for assessment. In the meantime, the patient should be advised to stick to a sugar-free diet. In the clinic we try to assess whether these patients are in urgent need of insulin (weight loss, ketones, high blood sugar). In most cases, there is no need for panic and we simply show them how to monitor their own blood glucose, aiming at results below 8 mmol/l.

Incidentally we are fortunate in having a single obstetrician who takes on all diabetic patients. This enables us to work as a partnership in joint clinics. It has been shown that specialist centres with this arrangement have a lower perinatal mortality for babies of diabetic mothers. If all the obstetricians in a maternity unit try to manage diabetes, there can be no joint clinic and communication between diabetologist, obstetrician and patient is often at risk.

Of the patients with impaired glucose tolerance, approximately 25% end up needing insulin to control blood glucose although they may not strictly speaking have diabetes according to WHO criteria. We usually apply the 30% rule:

30% continue to have raised glucose levels immediately after delivery.
30% regain normal glucose tolerance but go on to develop diabetes at some later stage in their life.
30% never develop diabetes unless they become pregnant again.
10% we do not know what happens to these people.

The large majority of these patients have NIDDM. Those that happen to develop IDDM during pregnancy need to be identified and start insulin straight away.

For your information, I enclose a copy of our Guidelines for Gestational Diabetes, which were put together by our obstetrician, diabetologist and clinical biochemist.

Yours sincerely

Figure 8.2

Guidelines for the management of gestational diabetes

These are intended as guidelines only. Please discuss individual circumstances with the Obstetric/Diabetic Clinic if you have any queries.

Identification of cases for screening

Patients should have a glucose load test if they fall into the following groups:

1. Previous gestational diabetes
2. Previous large baby (> 4.5 kg at term)
3. Previous unexplained stillbirth
4. Maternal family history of diabetes in parents or siblings
5. Gross maternal obesity (> 100 kg or marked central obesity)

Initial screening is carried out at booking. Repeat at 28 weeks if initial screen negative.

In addition, screening by glucose load is indicated if the following conditions develop during pregnancy:

1. Glycosuria of + or more on more than one occasion
2. Large for gestational age   *confirmed clinically*
3. Polyhydramnios   *by Consultant or scan*

Notes:

1. In some circumstances, previous gestational diabetes may merit proceeding straight to a full GTT (e.g. no record of a normal GTT after the previous pregnancy) – discuss preference with Consultant
2. If glycosuria persists after a normal GLT or GTT, it is not usually appropriate to retest unless there is another new indication, e.g. large for dates
3. Useful telephone numbers   (ensure that patient has these)

      Diabetes Centre
      Antenatal Assessment Unit
      Biochemistry Department

Method for glucose load test (GLT)

50g glucose is administered orally, irrespective of the time of the last meal. Blood glucose is measured exactly 60 minutes later.

If blood glucose is >7.5 mmol/l, further investigation is needed.

For patients less than 32 weeks gestation arrange a formal GTT with Biochemistry Department as soon as possible.

After 32 weeks gestation it may be more important to take action before a GTT appointment becomes available. Therefore in patients over 32 weeks, contact the Antenatal Assessment Unit (AAU) immediately who will arrange further investigation.

NB   A GLT is a screening test only. A raised GLT is NOT diagnostic of gestational diabetes.

Action in the event of an abnormal glucose tolerance test

NB   In pregnancy we take the following to be abnormal:

Fasting level > 6 mmol/l or two-hour level > 9 mmol/l

The Biochemistry Department will inform the Diabetes Centre. Patients will be seen in the next joint Obstetric/Diabetic Clinic in AAU. If the GTT was performed for some reason elsewhere, refer the result straight to the Diabetes Centre for further action.

ROUTINE CARE IN DIABETIC PREGNANCY

Pre-pregnancy

Pre-pregnancy care for diabetic women is not always possible but where it is ensure that good control of blood glucose levels (with an HbA1c <7.5%) is established prior to conception.

Advise women about the possibility of progression of eye and kidney disease.

Basis of management during pregnancy

1. Sugar-free diet
2. Home blood glucose monitoring. **All tests should ideally be in the range 4–7 mmol/l.** *Occasional* results of 7–9 are acceptable but the Diabetes team will advise individually.
3. Levels which are *frequently* in the range 7–9 mmol/l may require insulin.
4. Increased fetal surveillance – growth, liquor, movements and fetal monitoring. Delivery timing and route decided individually.

At and after delivery

Advise Paediatrician
Advise Diabetes Team – in labour or after delivery
Only patients on insulin antenatally require it in labour
Postnatal – insulin not normally required: Diabetes Team will advise
Discontinue home monitoring, resume normal diet

All patients with gestational diabetes should have a full GTT booked for six weeks post partum and an appointment made for the Obstetric/Diabetic Clinic for eight weeks to review results. Arrange this before discharge as it must not be missed.

First trimester

Early booking is advisable. Most diabetic mothers should have a dating scan at eight to ten weeks.

COMMANDMENT
Refer early for joint consultant care

It is important to continue emphasis on maintaining the best possible control. The following aspects of management should be discussed fully with the woman and educational literature provided to reinforce the messages:

■ Blood glucose monitoring
■ Insulin adjustment
■ Diet
■ Risk of hypos (and implications for driving, Glucagon use)
■ Access to specialist nurses
■ The diabetic clinic should be visited at least every four weeks. HbA1c should be tested on each visit, eyes should be checked for retinopathy, and blood pressure recorded

COMMANDMENT

Give individual dietary advice

COMMANDMENT

Warn the patient that diabetic pregnancies need close observation, and that hospital admission is a common price to pay for good care

Second trimester

Care during the second trimester has two main components, obstetric care and diabetic care.

Obstetric care

This follows the same pattern as care for non-diabetic women. In addition to the monthly antenatal visit, the mother will have blood taken for alphafetoprotein testing at 16 weeks and an anomaly scan at around 20 weeks. Other tests, such as amniocentesis, will be offered to diabetic women under the same criteria as would apply to non-diabetic women.

Diabetic care

The emphasis on good control of blood glucose continues. Women should also have their eyes checked for retinopathy.

Third trimester

The mother

As the pregnancy progresses, the mother will find that her insulin requirement increases. This will have to be observed closely and her doses of insulin adjusted as necessary.

Because of the increased incidence of pre-eclampsia in diabetic mothers, blood pressure will have to be tested more frequently than in other women and urine testing for protein-uria will also have to be regular.

Retinopathy should be screened for and its development monitored.

The fetus

Because of the risk of fetal macrosomia, serial growth scans are usually offered from 26 weeks.

Cardiotocograph monitoring of the fetus will be carried out weekly from 32 weeks.

Delivery

Ideally, the woman should be allowed to go into labour spontaneously shortly before term. However, most labours are likely to be induced at 38 to 39 weeks if all is going well. Caesarean section should be performed only for obstetric indications but women should be given some psychological preparation for the likelihood of this form of delivery as they are at much higher risk of caesarean section than the pregnant population at large.

All women with diabetes will be encouraged strongly to give birth in a consultant unit with appropriate facilities to assist both mother and baby. The mother will need an insulin/glucose infusion during labour and the baby will require continuous CTG monitoring.

If early delivery is necessary, steroids should be given prior to delivery. This helps the lungs to mature and reduces the risk of respiratory distress syndrome.

COMMANDMENT

Let the mother labour spontaneously at term or just before. Unless the baby is very large, a normal delivery is the best option

Post delivery

Newborn babies are likely to have trouble in stabilising their blood sugar levels once they are physiologically independent of the placenta. Most new babies of diabetic mothers will spend some time (usually 24 to 48 hours) in the Special Care Baby Unit until this problem resolves. The mother's insulin requirements will reduce dramatically after the birth of her baby. Insulin doses will need to be modified accordingly and are likely to return to pre-pregnancy levels. If the mother is breastfeeding her baby, she will need to be careful to ensure that her carbohydrate intake is sufficient.

COMMANDMENT

Observe both mother and baby closely during the immediate postnatal period. Adjust both diet and insulin dosage if the mother breastfeeds the baby

Once mother and baby have returned home, a visit by the diabetes specialist nurse should be arranged.

PREGNANCY IN WOMEN WITH NIDDM

As many people put off having children till they are older, a number will already have NIDDM. Those whose diabetes is managed by diet alone should simply monitor their blood glucose and await developments. Those who are taking sulphonylureas should stop as these may cross the placenta and cause an even larger baby.

DIABETES OUT OF ROUTINE

9

Diabetes is much easier to control when life is running along a clear path and many people with diabetes arrange to keep their lives well ordered to avoid uncertainty and difficult decisions. Long term survivors of diabetes often ascribe their achievement to maintaining a rigid discipline for 50 years or more with regular injections and meal times. Others manage the almost impossible task of incorporating well-controlled diabetes into a varied and disorganised life, though sadly these people are in a minority.

Even the more rigid types cannot escape the unexpected. Destabilisation can be caused by illness, family upsets or changes at work. Holidays and foreign travel are probably the most common events to break routine and the correspondence columns of journals for diabetic patients are full of questions about crossing time zones and coping with foreign food and meal times. This short chapter is not intended to give simplistic solutions to the questions you will be asked. However, in the spirit of the book, it should supply a strategy for dealing with them.

INTERCURRENT ILLNESS

At the onset of diabetes, it is often impressed on patients that soon after an insulin injection, they must always eat food to avoid the alarming experience of hypoglycaemia. There is a logical but false corollary that a patient who stops eating does not need insulin. At the onset of ketoacidosis, there may be loss of appetite and nausea and a patient may deprive him or herself of insulin, the one prerequisite for recovery. On rare occasions a doctor will reinforce this dangerous advice with potentially fatal consequences. In fact during most illnesses, patients need more rather than less insulin.

The rules for IDDs are given in Figure 9.1

Since most IDDs are able to measure blood glucose and adjust their insulin, they already have the tools for coping with illness, up to the point when intravenous fluid is needed. However NIDDs are limited in their scope for reacting to an increase in their insulin requirements. In hospital, it is easy

Figure 9.1

Insulin use during illness

DURING AN ILLNESS:

■   **DO NOT** stop insulin, simply because you stop eating

■   **CHECK** blood glucose **MORE FREQUENTLY** than usual – at least four times daily

■   If the results are high, **INCREASE** insulin and consider giving extra doses of short-acting insulin

■   **DRINK PLENTY** of fluids – aim at two litres (four pints) a day

■   Vomiting is a **SERIOUS** sign and usually requires hospital admission for intravenous fluids

■   **CHECK** urine for ketones. Heavy ketonuria is an indication for hospital admission

---

to give insulin on a short term basis. At home a GP without direct access to a specialist nurse might find it difficult to start insulin at short notice for the duration of the illness. In practice, most NIDDs seem to get away with a few days of hyperglycaemia and in the real world, insulin is not usually necessary during such ailments as a bad cold or an infection which responds to antibiotics. However, this is an unstable situation and if hyperglycaemia causes symptoms, or if there is vomiting, insulin and intravenous fluid will be needed.

SURGERY AND MAJOR INVESTIGATIONS

Most hospitals have protocols for the management of IDDM and NIDDM during surgical procedures. These consist of intravenous insulin, using a sliding scale for patients who are taking "nil by mouth".

Investigations which demand a fasting subject, such as gastroscopy and barium studies, can be perplexing for patients on insulin. If the procedure is to be first on a morning list, you and your patient should be able to work out a plan. Even this may be difficult in those patients who produce ketones after any delay in their morning insulin. If the test is scheduled later in the day, it may be necessary to contact those responsible and consider a brief in-patient stay to provide intravenous insulin and glucose for the period of fasting. In these days of bed shortages, arrangements need to be made in good time to avoid postponement.

As a general rule, patients on tablets for their diabetes can cope with a few hours of fasting. This becomes even safer if they can monitor the situation by testing their blood glucose.

SPORT

There are plenty of role models for young people with diabetes who wish to take part in nearly all sporting activities up to the highest level. Understandably strict conditions are placed on people with diabetes who participate in high risk sports such as scuba diving, parachute jumping and motor racing. Hypoglycaemia can make swimming dangerous, and patients should be given advice about the danger of swimming on their own.

Sports which involve extra energy expenditure increase the risk of hypoglycaemia. Most IDDs take the precaution of eating high energy food such as a Mars Bar before such activity and keeping glucose tablets or Lucozade available to correct a hypo. This approach has two drawbacks:

■   The sport has to be played on a full stomach
■   Regular exercise and hence extra calorie intake causes weight increase

The preferred option is to reduce insulin dose before exercise, thereby avoiding the need for extra food. This approach requires dedication and repeated blood glucose measurements to discover the correct dose reduction for a particular activity. The flexibility of the basal/bolus regimen simplifies dose adjustments.

HOLIDAYS AND TRAVEL

It would be nice to think that a holiday from work could also be a holiday from diabetes. Unfortunately change of diet, different meal times, altered energy output and extra alcohol all conspire against this dream. Thus more thought has to go into diabetes on holiday than in a routine week at the office. If a patient seeks advice, try to clarify the questions and together work out solutions.

Lengthy flights can be a problem with the risk of delays and crossing time zones. IDDs have to keep the full diabetic kit with their hand luggage. Food is easy to obtain during air travel and time changes can be overcome by giving short acting insulin before meals which usually appear every four to six hours. Blood glucose should be measured before each dose of insulin.

EATING OUT AND ALCOHOL

It should not be difficult to delay insulin dose and adjust it if necessary. Pen injectors and basal/bolus regimens both make this easier.

People with diabetes often receive gratuitous and inaccurate advice from the general public. For example, there is a misconception that diabetes and alcohol do not mix. In fact there is evidence that those who drink in moderation achieve better metabolic control than teetotallers. Alcohol does induce symptoms similar to those of neuroglycopenia and large doses of alcohol blunt the counter regulatory release of glucose from the liver. However, in practice these obstacles rarely lead to difficulties. People respond individually to a particular combination of alcohol in various guises accompanied by an intemperate amount of food. Suggest to patients who seek advice on rich food and alcohol that they make scientific sense out of the metabolic turmoil, by carrying out a "test meal" to reproduce the intake of food and drink. They will need a sober collaborator to carry out regular blood glucose measurements. In most cases the hyperglycaemic effect of food will overcome the hypoglycaemic action of alcohol but the experiment will provide useful information.

BEREAVEMENT, DIVORCE

Any tragic life event causes a disturbance in metabolic control. There is no evidence that the rise in blood glucose is due to excess output of adrenaline or other anti-insulin hormones, so the explanation must lie in behavioural factors. If life is dominated by a major tragedy, it is hard to devote to diabetes the attention it demands. People sometimes need permission to allow their diabetes to come low on their list of priorities during a time of personal crisis.

COMPLICATIONS

DIABETIC EYE DISEASE

10

NATURAL HISTORY

Everyone with diabetes has a fear of blindness.

> Christine is an intelligent, energetic professional woman whose diabetes was poorly controlled on tablets. She was worried about her high sugar levels but strongly resisted starting insulin treatment. She reminded me that her father had gone blind and lost his legs shortly after he was put onto insulin. She feared that the same fate would befall her.

In fact only 2% of the diabetic population ever go blind and this figure is bound to fall as result of energetic screening and treatment. However, diabetes is still quoted as the most common cause of blindness in people of working age, and it accounts for 20% of registrations in the age group 16 to 65 years.

**Dr AJC Pickering,
The Village Surgery**

Dear Charles

I'd appreciate you being able to see Sarah quite soon for counselling and surveillance of her diabetic retinopathy.

She is an intelligent, 19 year old student who developed diabetes when she was 12. She takes Human Mixtard 30 Pen twice daily and controls her blood sugar admirably as evidenced by blood sugars of 4 to 9 mmol/l and an HbA1c of 7% or so. She attends our miniclinic regularly and is free from any other problems. Her maternal uncle had diabetes and went blind at 42, so she is particularly sensitive to this complication. Her only other medical contact with us is for contraception - she takes Mercilon.

At our last clinic we dutifully dilated her pupils and I was concerned to see that she had in the preceding six months developed a cluster of microaneurysms between the disc and the fovea on the right. The left eye seems to be fine.

Sarah was understandably upset. She is anxious that she might follow in her uncle's footsteps and feels cheated that her years of careful control do not seem to have paid off. She asked about the contribution of the oral contraceptive to diabetic complications and about eye disease in pregnancy as she expects to marry in two years, after finishing her studies.

Do you think you might be able to see her with a view to counselling and let me know of your discussions for my own education?

Yours sincerely

Tony

RETINOPATHY

Retinopathy is one of the three classical complications of diabetes (together with nephropathy and neuropathy). All three are specific to diabetes and result from changes in the small blood vessels which may lead on to devastating problems for the patient. IDDs and NIDDs usually have a different pattern to their retinal changes and are considered separately.

Checking patients' eyes for retinopathy

GENERAL PRINCIPLES

Check visual acuity using a Snellen chart (with distance glasses, if worn, or a pinhole test). See pp 119–139.

Check fundi for signs of retinopathy. Dilate pupils with short-acting mydriatic, e.g. tropicamide. Use an ophthalmoscope with a bright light source.

Check the lens for cataracts. This can be done by looking at the eye from 6 inches (15 cm) using a + 8 (approximately) lens on the ophthalmoscope. With this process, any cataract will appear as a silhouette against the red reflex of the retina.

If visual acuity is reduced, but there is no sign of retinopathy, refer to optician. If there are signs of retinopathy, refer to ophthalmologist. If in doubt, refer.

Acknowledgement: these colour pictures are reproduced by kind permission of Prof. E. M. Kohner, Hammersmith Hospital, London.

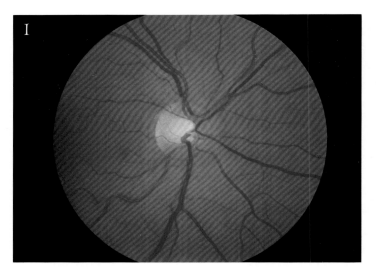

1. Normal retina. This picture shows a normal disc at centre. To the left, you can see part of the macula (or fovea), an area usually devoid of blood vessels.

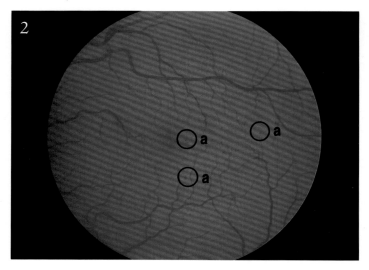

2. Mild background retinopathy. This centres on the macula (fovea). If you look closely, you will see a handful of microaneurysms which look like minute pink dots: some of these are marked (a). Refer to ophthalmologist.

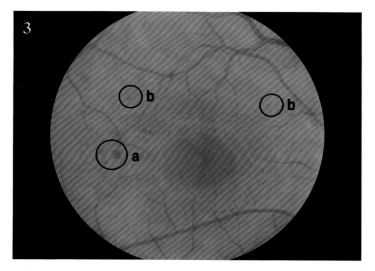

3. Mild background retinopathy, but showing dot and blot retinal haemorrhages (a) and some typical scattered microaneurysms (b). Refer to ophthalmologist.

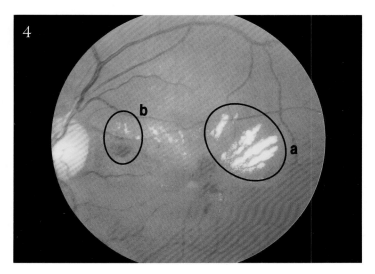

4. Maculopathy, at an advanced stage, with some streaks of hard exudate (a) almost surrounding the macula and another to the right of the disc, close to a blot haemorrhage (b). This degree of disease will be very difficult to treat with laser therapy. Urgent referral to ophthalmologist.

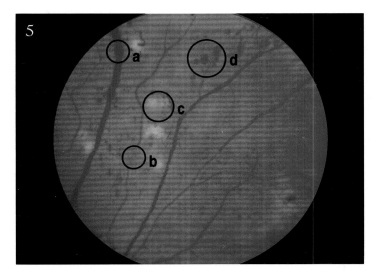

5. Preproliferative retinopathy with venous beading (a), intraretinal microvascular abnormalities (b), cotton wool spots (c), and clusters of haemorrhage (d). Urgent referral to ophthalmologist.

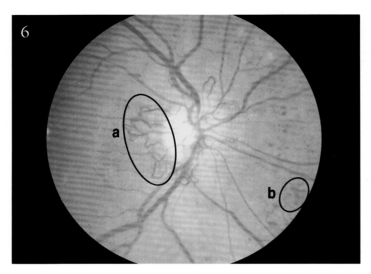

6. Severe proliferative retinopathy. An arcade of new vessels (a) encircling the disc. Some of these may be growing forward, but this can best be seen using a slit lamp. There are nasty retinal haemorrhages (b). Very urgent referral to ophthalmologist.

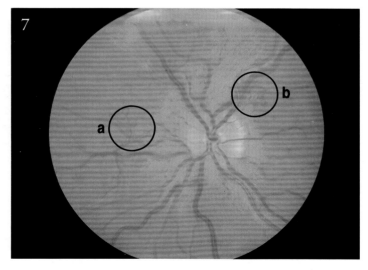

7. New vessels everywhere: clusters are clearly seen at (a) and (b). Very urgent referral to ophthalmologist.

Dr Charles Fox, The Diabetes Centre,
District General Hospital

Dear Tony,
    I agree that this is one of the heart-rending aspects
of diabetes care. At least Sarah was told the bad news by someone who
knew her well and was aware of the background (a real spin off of a
mini-clinic). I have just had the same experience in the Young Adult Clinic.
Ironically we had been talking about the DCCT in our discussion group and
had probably been doing a bit of brainwashing about the importance of
good control. The young patients had therefore focused on the question of
complications and were all a bit anxious about having their eyes examined. I
was congratulating Jane on her customary HbA1c below 7% and had said
that I had better check her eyes to be on the safe side. I had a strong
sense of disbelief when I saw a cluster of microaneurysms in each eye. I
had time to prepare what I would say but I knew I had a long session
ahead of me, dealing with Jane's indignation.
    I suppose we all tend to over-simplify biological data and need to
remember (and tell our patients) that good control reduces but does not
abolish the risk of complications. The other side of the coin is that many
patients who live happily with appalling control for many years seem to
be spared the ravages of diabetes. In the DCCT, about one in 15 patients
in the tight control group had a worsening of retinopathy during the
study while comparable figures for the poor control group were around
one in four.
    Many studies have used multivariate analysis to look for other non-
diabetic associations with the presence of complications. There have been
some interesting findings (e.g. tall people and drinkers of alcohol seem to
have protection against retinopathy and neuropathy), but there has been no
suggestion that the oral contraceptive pill is a risk factor. Pregnancy is a bit
different, in that about 10% of pregnant women with diabetes develop an
active form of retinopathy which may require repeated laser therapy
throughout the time of pregnancy and into the first few months of the puer-
perium. I have not seen any proven explanation for this. It is usually put
down to "hormones" but I wonder if it is not a manifestation of the well-
recognised phenomenon that a sudden improvement in metabolic control may
lead to a transient worsening in retinopathy.
    It is interesting that Sarah has personal experience of devastating
diabetic complications. This emphasises the importance of taking a full
family history when diabetes is first diagnosed. Her uncle must have been a
significant figure in her childhood and Sarah's parents must have this negative model of diabetes in their minds. There is also the question of whether
genetic factors govern the risk of diabetic complications. Some studies have
purported to show this but it is generally felt that they were too small to be
valid and that there are no independent genetic risk factors which make one

diabetic family more or less likely to get problems. Of course behavioural traits may be inherited but that is a different matter.

I have put off counselling till last – perhaps we all need psychological help in coping with these distressing cases. I will certainly put aside a lot of time to see Sarah and will try to get in tune with her own feelings. She may feel resentful that despite her best efforts she has run into trouble but at least she should be spared the guilt that many people in her position experience. I will find out what she feels about her uncle. Families can be quite harsh critics and he might even have been victimised and blamed for causing his own blindness by not taking his diabetes seriously. I might even ask Sarah if she realises that you were upset to be the person who broke the bad news about her "micros". Having heard about her own feelings and beliefs, I will carry out what has been called "educational counselling" with an attempt to get the whole problem in perspective. She may wish to know more about the process of retinopathy and what can be done to prevent it. In fact I would judge that there is only a minute chance of Sarah going blind in the future.

Yours sincerely

Retinopathy in IDDM

As a rule, the first signs of retinopathy are not seen in IDDM until at least five years after diagnosis, but there are rare exceptions which lodge in the memory and oblige us to look in the eyes of all patients with diabetes. The retinal changes in IDDM usually develop in a step-wise manner, which makes it easy to stage the process:

1. Background changes
2. Macular changes
3. Pre-proliferative changes
4. Proliferative retinopathy
5. End stage disease

Background changes

These are defined as abnormalities in the retina due to diabetes which are no threat to vision. They do not require laser therapy.

The earliest reliable sign of diabetic retinopathy is the *microaneurysm* (or "micro"). The micro is a tiny blemish the size of a pinprick which may take a bit of finding – even with dilated pupils. One or two micros can often be seen in each eye without any other evidence of diabetic retinopathy. When there are more than ten micros in an eye, however, there is a high chance of finding other changes such as small retinal haemorrhages and scattered hard exudates. As long as these changes do not encroach on the macula, they do not threaten vision and can be classified as background changes.

COMMANDMENT

If, with dilated pupils, you can see more than ten microaneurysms, search hard for other problems e.g. disc new vessels or macular changes

Macular changes

Abnormalities which would be innocent elsewhere in the retina may be of serious significance if close to the macula, which is responsible for all our high-definition vision. Thus a cluster of micros or hard exudates at the posterior pole may herald the appearance of macular oedema. These appearances require referral to an ophthalmologist.

Pre-proliferative change

This is a state of great activity, in which a spectrum of different lesions is seen. These include cotton wool spots (sometimes known as soft exudates), intra-retinal microvascular abnormalities, and "dot and blot" retinal haemorrhages. This stage merges imperceptibly into the next.

Proliferative retinopathy

This involves the appearance of new blood vessels which may be either close to the optic disc or at the periphery of the retina. Either way they are liable to bleed, leading to a haemorrhage into the vitreous body (the jelly of the eye) and serious loss of vision, particularly if the macula is obscured.

End stage disease

Haemorrhage and new vessels are replaced by opaque fibrous tissue which also contracts and leads to retinal detachment. New vessels can also invade the filtration angle and cause a painful irreversible glaucoma. At this stage it may be necessary to enucleate the eye to relieve pain.

Retinopathy in NIDDM

This is usually a less dramatic process than the horrendous series of events detailed above. The changes tend to be clustered around the macula and often cause a mild reduction in visual acuity before anyone realises that there is a problem. Many old people with diabetic retinopathy have been given a series of costly new spectacles and the true nature of the problem has been mistaken for "old age" or cataract. Elderly people with diabetes are likely to suffer other illnesses and disabilities. A relatively minor visual loss may compound their

Dr AJC Pickering,
The Village Surgery

Dear Charles

I would be grateful for your help with James Parker, a 71 year old retired engineer, who has quite marked retinopathy. He presented recently with polyuria and polydipsia, was found to have a high blood sugar and started on dietary control. As part of our monthly review of new NIDDs we invited him to our diabetic clinic for a "baseline" check.

Although I was aware that NIDDs can have retinopathy at presentation, I was shocked to find extensive changes, microaneurysms in profusion and hard exudates adjacent to both foveas but in particular cotton wool spots around the left disc at about 3 o'clock. I guess this constitutes pre-proliferative retinopathy.

His visual acuity is 6/9 on the left and 6/6 on the right, using his corrective lenses.

His blood sugar is coming slowly under control, now 11-15 mmol/l having been 24+ mmol/l at diagnosis. He has managed in the last six weeks to shed some 5 kg in weight from a fairly modest 92 kg (BMI 30). I suspect he has reached the limit of dietary control and we shall have to start him on oral hypoglycaemics in addition to diet.

Apart from the request for your expert assessment of his eye disease, I would value your comments on the following:

- *is laser therapy painful?*
- *is it known to benefit the elderly?*
- *what is likely to happen to his eye disease as we bring the glucose under control still further; that is, is he in the same category in this respect as folk whose retinopathy accelerates on starting insulin? Is the trigger the therapy or the effect on blood glucose?*

Thank you, as ever, for your help.

Yours sincerely

Tony

**Dr Charles Fox, The Diabetes Centre,
District General Hospital**

Dear Tony

I enjoyed meeting James in the new patient clinic. We normally ask newly diagnosed NIDDs to come to a series of information sessions before they actually get to see a doctor. This gives them the information they need plus a bit of group support and avoids the need for the doctor to have to take on a major educational role. Because of worries about his eyes, James bypassed this system but would like to find out more about diabetes and he and his wife Nora will be coming along to the sessions over the next few weeks. He will be a valuable contributor to the session on complications.

It does come as a shock when you find extensive retinopathy in a newly diagnosed patient. One of the hospital switchboard operators turned up in our new patient clinic a few years ago complaining that she could not see well enough to do her job. She had end stage and untreatable retinopathy and had spent a fortune on different spectacles over the previous two years. Most opticians can be relied upon to detect retinal disease, but unfortunately she had been to someone who felt that a change of glasses would always do the trick. Had she been seen by us earlier, I am sure laser would have preserved useful vision.

James certainly has advanced retinopathy as you describe. The cotton wool spots do suggest that he may go on to develop new vessels in his left eye, but the main immediate worry is the presence of hard exudates close to the fovea (I call it macula) in both eyes. I have asked our ophthalmologist to see him within a month and I am sure she will apply the laser to try and clear up the oedema that must underlie these florid exudates.

James repeated your questions about the discomfort caused by laser therapy and its effectiveness in older people. I didn't get the impression that he was particularly anxious but, like most engineers, he has a pretty mechanistic approach to medical problems. I tried to get across the idea that human eyes are not printed circuits and that people vary in their response to laser therapy. In fact the treatment is a pretty atraumatic experience, partly because of the communication skills of our ophthalmologist who explains what she is going to do and inspires great confidence. I have told James that he will have drops to dilate his pupil to give a clear view and anaesthetic drops so that he can tolerate the contact lens that will be applied to his eye to focus the laser beam. He will experience a bright flash with each application but this is not painful except in people who have had repeated treatment sessions. Because of the mydriatic, he will have to get a lift home and may feel a bit of an ache in his eye a few hours after treatment.

Laser is very effective in old people especially if they have early macular changes which respond to a few applications of laser. Old people are more likely to have cataract which can make it difficult both to identify and treat retinal disease. We are usually keen for our patients to have their cataracts removed so that we can see what is going on in the retina. James has very clear lenses as confirmed by his good visual acuities and he will cooperate well with the laser treatment so I am sure there will be no problems. Although his retinopathy is already advanced, his macula is spared and, though he may need several laser sessions, the prognosis for his vision is reasonably good.

He is now feeling a lot better with sugars in the low teens, but I feel he will probably need some additional help. In view of his "modest" 87 kg, he would be a good candidate for metformin starting at 500 mg tds. I have warned about the side-effects and given him our leaflet about metformin. It is true that, in people with longstanding poor control, a sudden improvement in blood sugars can paradoxically increase the activity in the retina for six to twelve months, after which the benefits of good control reassert themselves. This is seen in younger people with IDDM, and I don't think this would happen in NIDDM where retinopathy is a more insidious process, often associated with retinal ischaemia.

Yours sincerely

disabilities and prevent them from leading an independent existence.

Unlike IDDs, people with NIDDM frequently have some degree of retinopathy at the time of diagnosis. This is usually only at the background stage but, from time to time, people turn up for the first time in the diabetic clinic with retinal disease which is past the stage at which laser therapy will help. The UKPDS has accumulated valuable information about the prevalence of retinal disease in NIDDM (see Figure 10.1).

Macular changes

People with NIDDM may show the same progression of retinal disease as described above for IDDM. However, it usually starts

Figure 10.1

Proportion of patients with retinopathy (defined as microaneurysms in both eyes or more severe retinopathy in one eye) as identified by the UKPDS

Diagnosis	18%
3 yrs	26%
6 yrs	34%
9 yrs	40%
12 yrs	53%

with a few hard exudates and microaneurysms around the macula. Sometimes the changes look innocent but because of their position, they may cause visual failure. It is particularly important to refer these patients to an ophthalmologist since a few bursts of laser therapy are often all that is needed to eradicate the problem.

COMMANDMENT

Take seriously any changes close to the macula, however innocent they may appear. They could cause loss of vision

Factors influencing the development of retinopathy

The definitive answer to the relationship between metabolic control and the development of retinopathy has come from the DCCT (see Chapter 3). This showed that in the group with "tight" control (HbA1c around 7.1%) retinopathy progressed much more slowly than in the group with less good control (HbA1c of 9.5%).

The DCCT was carried out in a large group of well-motivated patients with IDDM. It is not known whether the findings can be applied to NIDDM. This question will be answered by the UKPDS which is due to be analysed in 1998. Retinopathy is related to the presence of other complications, particularly nephropathy. This simply reflects that both are manifestations of the same process, namely disease of small blood vessels.

Some published work has suggested that cigarette smoking and raised blood pressure are independent risk factors for developing retinopathy, but the evidence is not conclusive.

OTHER EYE PROBLEMS THAT MAY BE RELATED TO DIABETES

Cataracts

There is a rare form of cataract which results from a high blood glucose and may occur in young people with longstanding poor diabetic control. These were seen 10 or 20 years ago but are now a thing of the past.

Ordinary "senile" cataracts are much more common in people with diabetes and they occur at an earlier age. They can be treated in the same way with lens implants if necessary.

Glaucoma

Patients with proliferative retinopathy may develop an unpleasant form of painful glaucoma due to new vessels blocking up the filtration angle.

Retinal vein thrombosis

This process may affect either the central vein in the retina or one of the branch veins draining a quadrant of the retinal

**Dr AJC Pickering,
The Village Surgery**

Dear Charles

Could you advise, in general terms, on how we might better help people whose sight is deteriorating. I have in mind 68 year old Ahmed Khan who was diagnosed with diabetes ten years ago and has been passably well controlled on glibenclamide (HbA1c around 9%). Last year he suffered a retinal haemorrhage and was found inter alia to have glaucoma (in annual checks he had been noted to have only background retinopathy). Since then he has developed progressive and intractable eye pain and diminishing acuity.

For obvious reasons he is effectively housebound. He seems to have a retarded depression, being increasingly insouciant and preferring to sit in his chair all day. His wife, who has hypertension, obesity and nasty arthritis of the knees, tells me that he has stopped his favourite pastime of gardening and talks increasingly of dying. He complains of little but I gather he gets jolly angry at meal times when he has trouble cutting up food, and he hates being shaved by his wife.

He used to watch lots of sport on the television and read one or two books a week from the town library.

He has not taken up my suggestions of contact with the RNIB and although registered partially sighted has declined an offer to attend the visual aids unit for assistance. He does not accept my suggestion that he is depressed and refuses to contemplate antidepressants.

Can you give me some guidance on the sort of approach I might take with him?

Yours sincerely

Tony

TEACHING POINT

The normal form of glaucoma (primary open angle) is twice as common in people with diabetes. The reason for this is not known

Dr Charles Fox, The Diabetes Centre,
District General Hospital

Dear Tony

You tell the sad story of a previously active elderly man whose life has been diminished by blindness due to diabetes. The retinal haemorrhage was presumably from an occult diabetic new vessel which was not detected at previous screening. I was not clear why Ahmed had glaucoma. I assume this is the chronic simple variety which is unrelated to diabetes, but commonly leads to blindness in older people. On the other hand, diabetic new vessel disease may infiltrate the filtration angle and cause glaucoma which leads to intractable pain. Presumably, you have exhausted ways of retrieving in some degree his visual failure?

Ahmed would be helped by loss counselling to help him acknowledge the problem and think of ways of rebuilding his life in terms of his handicap. I do not have easy access to anyone who might help but I heard you were thinking of employing a counsellor in your practice.

Ahmed has lost his sense of enjoyment, has lost his energy and suffers morbid thoughts, all clear evidence of depression. Reactive depression responds perfectly well to antidepressant therapy. If his painful eye keeps him awake, you could always suggest that an antidepressant might help him get off to sleep. I have to admit that this sort of ploy seldom works and such patients always seem to experience unacceptable side-effects.

Yours sincerely

circulation. Central retinal vein occlusion (CRVO) causes sudden loss of central vision, sometimes with pain in the affected eye. The fundus looks congested with numerous retinal haemorrhages – rather as if a bomb had gone off inside the eye. Sometimes in younger patients the vision can recover over a few weeks. Patients with CRVO, whether associated with diabetes or not, may subsequently develop new vessels and require laser therapy.

Branch retinal vein occlusion leads to a visual field defect and the severity depends on whether the macula is involved, thus affecting central vision.

TEACHING POINT

Both central and branch vein occlusion are more common in diabetes but also occur in people with raised blood pressure, atheroma and chronic simple glaucoma

---

Ophthalmoplegia

This dramatic complication of diabetes is not uncommon and requires great diagnostic confidence and powers of re-assurance on the part of the doctor. It presents with sudden diplopia, often preceded by pain in the affected eye. The problem may affect any one of the three cranial nerves controlling eye movements. If you can remember which muscles are innervated by each cranial nerve, it is easy to work out which nerve is involved in the mononeuropathy (LR6S04). If this is indeed the diagnosis, there is nothing more to be done except wait patiently for re-innervation to take place. However, sudden onset of diplopia may sometimes result from a more sinister cause than diabetes.

If diabetes is the cause of the isolated nerve palsy, there will almost certainly be a full recovery in due course. It may take several months before the diplopia begins to improve and this period of waiting can be very frustrating for the patient, and strained for the doctor who has put his or her reputation on the line by promising that it will all get completely better.

Colour blindness

This is a common abnormality in the non-diabetic population. Ten per cent of men have some degree of red-green colour blindness.

Patients should be asked whether they have any problems differentiating between shades of colour and if there is any doubt this aspect of vision should be tested. Colour vision test cards come in books of different cards, all of which show different shades of colour in mosaic patterns. The range of cards in a book will test different variants of colour vision defects.

It may also be helpful to have patients read urine testing or blood testing sticks in front of you to show you whether their colour vision is likely to present problems with self-testing.

Refractive errors

It is common for newly diagnosed patients to complain that for the past few months they have had intermittent blurred vision. This is due to high sugar levels causing the lens to swell osmotically, thereby leading to myopia. Some patients notice that their refraction is very sensitive to changes in blood glucose concentration and they know that their levels are high when their vision is blurred.

TREATMENT

The treatment for diabetic retinopathy is laser therapy. When there are widespread aggressive changes in the fundi, patients may require thousands of laser applications over several treatment sessions, which are tiring for both the patient and the ophthalmologist. Older patients with no more than a few hard exudates close to the macula may only need a few dozen applications to eradicate the exudates and preserve their sight – and hence their independence. A successful laser therapist needs to be skilled technically but also needs to know when to apply the treatment. As a rule, ophthalmologists are treating patients earlier in the natural history of their disease. They have found that widespread therapy given just before new vessels develop reduces the total treatment needed. Even more striking is the response of a small exudate close to the macula which will disappear after a few bursts of laser, thus preserving visual acuity.

Vitrectomy

Surgery still has a place when the eye has serious retinal damage in the form of vitreous haemorrhages and fibrous tissue. When the vitreous body is opaque, it can be removed by a machine known in the trade as "the gobbler". At the same time any fibrous bands can be resected and detached retina stuck back onto the sclera. This last-ditch surgery is not usually effective, perhaps because patients are not referred early enough.

SCREENING

The Patients' Charter produced by the British Diabetic Association recommends that every person with diabetes has an eye check every year. In practice, it is unusual for insulin-dependent patients to develop any form of retinopathy within the first five years. However there are enough exceptions to make most diabetologists want to examine ALL patients

COMMANDMENT

Ensure that all patients with diabetes, especially IDDs of more than five years' standing and all NIDDs, have their retina checked by someone competent every year

annually. There is no harm in making patients feel that ophthalmoscopy is a routine procedure carried out at every annual review. It may not be necessary to use a mydriatic in young people with "clear eyes" and pupils that are naturally widely dilated.

Methods of screening

Visual acuity

This routine activity is often surprisingly difficult to organise. In the first place you need a well-lit (or internally lit) Snellen chart and a spot at six metres distance where the patient can stand. We had great difficulty finding a clear six metre run in the diabetic clinic, and the same might be true for a busy surgery. At first we had the chart on a swing door in a busy corridor which caused a few problems. We have now suspended the chart high up in a quiet corner of the clinic. It is possible to use a half size chart or a complicated system of mirrors, which reduces the distance to three metres.

Patients should be asked to bring distance glasses to the clinic. The right eye should be tested first, while the left is covered with a card. Patients should read down the chart and the tester should record the lowest line the patient can manage. If there are errors in the line, record as follows: 6/9 − 2. If the patient normally wears spectacles and forgot to bring them, the refractive error can be corrected using a pinhole. Having checked the right eye, cover this and test the left eye.

Fundoscopy

Ideally this should be done by a suitably trained doctor after the pupils have been dilated with a mydriatic. Tropicamide 1% has become routine. Like most eye drops, it stings for 10 to 20 seconds and takes up to 20 minutes to have its full effect.

Dr AJC Pickering,
The Village Surgery

Dear Charles

With my GP Tutor hat on I would like your opinion on some ideas for CME topics about diabetic eye disease.

My premise is that some GPs don't examine the optic fundi of their diabetic patients because they are scared of not recognising diabetic retinal pathology. They then make use of the other facilities for screening such as opticians or non-mydriatic photography or are much relieved when the patient attends having driven to the surgery, believing that they should not then dilate the pupils. My thesis is that we could usefully encourage an attitude of "all or none", that is definitely normal or refer. We should couple this with individual feedback so that GPs gradually come to recognise the features of retinopathy from a position of safety.

I understand the ophthalmologists have some rather clever models of eyes that one examines using an ophthalmoscope and in which the pathology can be changed rather as one might change a slide. Do you think we might organise a skills session using this system? I would imagine that we should repeat this every two years or so to reinforce the pattern recognition and allow those who had not attended to come along.

Certainly I feel the need for some sort of reassurance in this area and there are a lot of patients who for various reasons never get to the optician or the hospital, notably those who are housebound.

Yours sincerely

Tony

**Dr Charles Fox, The Diabetes Centre,
District General Hospital**

Dear Tony

Retinal screening is the hot potato of diabetes care. There are heavy artillery battles in the literature between supporters of the retinal camera and those who make use of the skills of local optometrists. Many GPs who run the best diabetic clinics in their own surgeries feel insecure about retinal examination. I suppose the guiding principle should be the provision of the system which is safest and most convenient for patients. If screening methods are not user-friendly, a low take-up rate will defeat the object of the exercise. Thus for patients who attend the hospital clinic, we try to combine retinal screening with the rest of the annual review. As the focus of diabetes care moves towards general practice, it seems logical to train GPs to carry out retinal screening with confidence. I agree that it should be simple to teach a doctor how to recognise a normal fundus and to organise a quick response for any patient who, in the GP's opinion, falls outside this category. Perhaps at this stage the retinal camera could be used to provide a permanent record of the abnormality and a report to the GP which would aid the teaching process.

It would be an interesting challenge to set up such a training scheme for GPs who are already running their own diabetic clinics. We know that practice nurses are performing many of the screening tasks in GP clinics. Would it be heresy to suggest that nurses might become rather good at wielding the ophthalmoscope? This would also get round the problem of GPs who were not keen to learn how to examine the fundus.

Yours sincerely

Tropicamide lasts two to three hours and it is not necessary to use reversing drops.

Retinal examination is not always easy and it may take some time for a doctor to be confident about the significance of any retinal abnormality. Of course it is easier for a doctor to recognise that there is some abnormality seen on fundoscopy, as opposed to having the experience to identify all the many different features of diabetic retinopathy.

Because of the difficulty of organising retinoscopy by trained doctors, many districts have organised alternative systems for carrying out this essential exercise. The usual arrangement is to train optometrists to carry out screening and refer patients with retinopathy directly to an eye specialist. Another system employs a retinal camera, usually using a single shot per eye to produce a Polaroid print. This can be reported by a qualified doctor or technician and has the advantage that a permanent record is available for future comparison.

There would probably not be a 100% take up, but the camera would always be available for patients of those GPs who did not take part.

Pitfalls of retinal screening

There are three possible reasons why retinal screening may fail to identify the patient who is developing serious disease of the retina:

1.   *Failure of the observer or screening system to identify the problem*

This can occur if the pupils are not fully dilated or the retinas are obscured by cataract. An experienced observer will insist on correcting these obstacles. Rarely, there may be significant disease limited to the periphery of the retina, which is outside the field of view of the retinal camera.

2.   *Rapid deterioration within the timespan of the next planned screening*

Once there is significant active retinopathy, the retina should be examined carefully every six months, rather than annually. There are two factors which are recognised to cause a sudden deterioration in retinopathy, namely pregnancy and a sudden improvement in diabetic control. Under these conditions, patients should be examined every two months.

3.   *Failure of the patient to attend the screening procedure*

This highlights the need to involve the patient in the screening process and to emphasise its importance. It may help to provide the patient with a written report which includes an invitation to return in 12 months for review.

EDUCATION POINT FOR PATIENTS

Retinotherapy does not usually cause noticeable loss of vision until it reaches an advanced stage. By then it may be too late to treat it with laser therapy. Regular screening by a qualified person means that treatment can be given at an earlier stage, which often makes the process simpler and quicker

FEET

Foot ulceration is a common cause of hospital admission amongst diabetic patients. In 1991, 6000 patients attending British diabetes clinics were surveyed. Over 2% had active foot ulcers and 2.5% were amputees. The risk of lower limb amputations is 15 times greater in diabetics compared to the non-diabetic population, and more than 50% of diabetic amputees lose the remaining leg within four years. In 1985, the cost of diabetic amputations was estimated at £13.4 million.

If only we might follow the biblical exhortation "For He shall give His angels charge over thee: to keep thee in all thy ways / They shall bear thee in thy hands: that thou shalt not hurt thy foot".

Teaching in medical school has focused traditionally on the disease of diabetes itself, with less emphasis on complications. We start our careers with little information about the cost, either to society or to the individual and family, of disease of the feet in diabetes. But everyone involved with diabetes care soon learns of the personal suffering this complication causes.

Foot care tends to be low on our list of clinical priorities. Doctors, nurses and people with diabetes often take the view that such things just happen. Thus an important element of managing the problem is the continuing education of both carers and patients.

PATHOLOGY AND SYMPTOMS

Diabetic foot problems stem from the twin pathological processes of neuropathy and ischaemia.

Neuropathy

Neuropathy may be painful or painless, and involve the sensory, motor or autonomic functions. As a rule, painless neuropathy is more of a worry than the painful variety, because severe destruction of the foot may occur before the patient seeks medical advice. An impaired nerve supply may damage muscles in the foot, producing "clawing" of the toes, while loss of subcutaneous tissue leads to extremely high pressures at certain points, most commonly under the head of the first metatarsal. The foot responds to the high pressure by laying down callus which, in turn, damages the underlying tissues and causes ulceration. Any break in the skin may be an entry site for infection which may fester without being noticed until it has reached an advanced stage.

COMMANDMENT
Examine the feet at least once a year

Any patient with numb feet should have regular checks by a skilled podiatrist who will treat any callus and advise about footwear.

Patients may describe "pins and needles", a "burning pain", "toothache in the foot" or excessive and abnormal sensation, particularly at night. Alcohol may exacerbate the symptoms.

Autonomic dysfunction in the foot causes decreased sweating, vascular calcification, overperfusion, arteriovenous shunting, increased bone absorption or oedema. It is an important factor in the development of ulcers and can occur at any stage in diabetes.

Ischaemia

Ischaemia causes pain which occurs initially on exertion (claudication), but may progress to pain at rest, and beyond – to critical ischaemia. The underlying atheroma may affect large or small vessels, or both. The level of arterial blockage is usually evident on careful inspection of the legs and feet, and by feeling for the peripheral pulses. A high block will lead to absent or feeble femoral pulses, with no distal pulses palpable. In such cases, intervention is more likely to succeed, though there is still the chance that co-existing arterial disease will frustrate the efforts of the vascular surgeon or the radiologist who attempts angioplasty. Management decisions are influenced by the degree of symptoms and level of ischaemia requiring emergency treatment.

Ischaemia is multifactorial and, consequently, difficult to treat. Smoking is a particular risk. The accelerated atherosclerosis accompanying the hyperlipidaemia so common in

CHECKLIST FOR IDENTIFYING THE FOOT AT RISK

1. **Previous foot ulcer**

2. **Reduced vibration sense**

3. **Impaired blood supply**

4. **Smoking and alcohol excess**

5. **Social deprivation**

6. **Structural abnormality of the foot**

Dr AJC Pickering,
The Village Surgery

Dear Charles

You may yet rue the day you encouraged mini-clinics, for after every one I seem to write to you. At least this time it is with an idea!

As a "gate-keeper" to the limited resources of NHS secondary care, I cannot reasonably send you every corn, callus, minor degree of neuropathy or minimal case of vascular damage for I would then surely overload the system. At the same time, I am aware that my failure to refer early enough may result later in an inevitable referral (by you) for amputation.

At which point along the progression between normality and extreme pathology does "care in the community" become a misnomer?

I realise there is no clear cut answer but could you suggest any guidelines?

Would it be possible to grade the degree of pathology on a scale from 1 to 5 and suggest a scoring system for referral? For example:

Loss of vibration sense distally	1
More than two calluses	2
Loss of vibration sense distally and proximally	3
Trophic ulcer	5
Cold feet	1
Absence of one foot pulse	2
Absence of both foot pulses	3
etc.	

Referral would be indicated at an aggregate score of, say, 5 or more.

I realise there is no research to establish such a formula, but I wonder if one might not be able to quantify the mental process that you, as an expert, use to judge the severity of foot pathology. One might perhaps refine the rating system over time, through audit.

What do you think?

Yours aye

Tony

**Dr Charles Fox, The Diabetes Centre,
District General Hospital**

Dear Tony

You know me well enough to predict that I would never be party to introducing a new scoring system (outside a research project). I don't have that sort of organised mind. However, your point is important and I agree that we need clear guidelines on when to act urgently over a particular diabetic foot problem. I agree too with your idea of a hierarchy of complications.

Anyone with diabetes and a foot problem, for example athlete's foot, ingrowing toenail or hallux valgus, warrants referral to podiatry.

I suggest the following qualitative approach to priority in treating foot problems:

Neuropathic	
Loss of vibration sense	Education
Callus or any deformity	Refer to podiatrist
Neuropathic ulcer	Refer to podiatrist and diabetologist
Infected ulcer	Urgent admission

Ischaemic	
No pulses, no pain	Education
No pulses, claudication	Refer to vascular surgeon
No pulses, rest pain + discoloration	Urgent referral to vascular surgeon
Gangrene/pre-gangrene	Urgent admission

If we set up a research project we will have to work out a quantitative system. The suggestions made depend on local services. Some centres identify patients with a "foot at risk" and provide them with intensive education. These patients are encouraged to bring themselves immediately to the podiatry department if they notice any deterioration in their feet.

Yours sincerely

COMMANDMENT

Be aware that painless neuropathy puts feet at risk and requires serious podiatry

diabetes may also play a part. Ischaemic heart disease and reduced cardiac output contribute to poor perfusion and may tip the balance between acceptable and critical ischaemia.

Vascular pain is suggested by claudication and rest pain unrelieved by walking. This is in contrast to neuropathic pain which is often nocturnal and may be relieved by activity. Vascular disease may be stable for years only to become severe quite suddenly, frequently as a result of heart failure.

Disease of both nervous and vascular systems may confuse the diagnosis and obscure the optimal treatment. Is the pain vascular or neurological? It is a worrisome combination and, if there is doubt in a serious case, angiography or Duplex Doppler studies and electromyography (EMG) will help to quantify each component of the pain.

EDUCATION

The challenge of assessing the correct educational approach is easier if the doctor knows the individual's backround and

COMMANDMENT

Examine the feet to educate both yourself and your patient

CHECKLIST
EXAMINATION OF THE FEET

1. **Observe colour and temperature**

2. **Check posterior tibial and dorsalis pedis pulses**

3. **Test with tuning fork on tip of big toe**

4. **Look carefully for corns, calluses, deformity**

5. **Check between toes for athlete's foot**

6. **Look at footwear**

Throughout this process, explain what you are doing and describe the findings

response to other problems. The task suits the primary health care team particularly well. The attitude of the "teacher", and a readiness to accept the patient as a responsible adult is fundamental to a successful educational outcome. It is in part a battle of wits and, as always, it feels good to win.

Listen, look and talk. The process of examination reinforces the importance we attach to foot care and provides an opportunity to explain and listen further. A team approach with the podiatrist as leader and team educator allows the delivery of an expert, consistent message.

Consultation skills are vital to an effective outcome. We have limited time, but we need to assess the patient's understanding of the issue and recruit him or her by sharing our conclusions and agreeing a cooperative strategy. Listening and an appropriate questioning style, involving open-ended questions as leaders and closed questions to focus on specific areas, may reveal the symptoms of pain or numbness.

Dr AJC Pickering,
The Village Surgery

Dear Charles

I have just finished a diabetic clinic in the practice and been forcibly reminded of a problem about which I would appreciate your views.

It seems that people with diabetes fall into one of three groups in respect of their feet: those with no risk factors (being of normal weight, non smokers and with normal sensation and pulses); those with established disease in their feet; and — if my experience today is anything to go by — the majority who have something minor amiss (some mix of loss of vibration sense, cold feet, poor microcirculation, absent pulses, calluses or deformed feet).

Within this group, there are a number of people who resist our "easy to follow" advice. Frankly, this is frustrating and irritating. I am puzzled by their poor compliance.

Our stance is to take the view that, having given them information in the right way, what happens is up to them. Is this nihilism? Another approach is to consider that the problem lies with us, in a failure to strike the right chord at the right time.

Have you any hints about the psychological approach to take?

Yours in frustration

Tony

There is evidence that good foot care can prevent foot complications and reduce amputation rates. Excellent leaflets are available from pharmaceutical companies and from hospital departments of podiatry.

It is worth checking that the patient does not take beta blockers and, when asking about smoking, explain its role in disease of the feet.

COMMANDMENT

Establish a close working link with
a podiatrist

**Dr Charles Fox, The Diabetes Centre,
District General Hospital**

Dear Tony

You are right to suppose that some sort of foot disease is common in patients attending a clinic for their annual review, particularly if your clinic population consists mainly of NIDDs who tend to be older. I agree that the big problem in foot education is persuading the patient that there is a problem. I often wonder whether shock tactics would make people take their feet more seriously. I could invite patients to join the ward round on diabetic feet – a weekly reminder of the mutilation diabetes can cause. As a rule, the people who treat their feet conscientiously have usually had direct experience that diabetes can maim. On the other hand, psychologists insist that fear is not a good motivator. Following a first amputation, patients do not always make sensible decisions about the preservation of their remaining leg.

Many of those with serious neuropathy lack sensation in their feet and can develop extensive ulceration without feeling any pain. If they also have poor vision, the first hint of trouble may be the smell from their damaged foot, infected with an anaerobic organism. I remember a policeman with neuropathy who walked around all day with a nail sticking through the sole of his shoe into his foot. He only discovered the nail when the ulcer was healed and he went to clean his shoes before returning to work. Apart from sensory loss, social deprivation is another major risk for neuropathic foot ulceration. Perhaps people lower down the social scale walk further, find it more difficult to rest their feet and have less suitable footwear.

To be effective, education must always start from the patients' standpoint, using their own perceptions and beliefs. Education must also be relevant and strike a chord. I always feel uncomfortable when I hear an "expert" advising young people with a short history of diabetes not to walk barefoot. When I examine a patient's feet, I try to explain in detail what I am doing and deal with each aspect in turn – pulse, sensation, footwear, deformities, callus etc. I try to explain gently what goes wrong in a "worst case scenario". The best bet is to refer your patient to a podiatrist with an interest in both education and diabetes, if you are lucky to have access to such an exemplary person.

This answer has focused on the classic case of the unconcerned patient with a nasty neuropathic foot ulcer. Ischaemic foot problems tend to cause more anxiety simply because they cause pain. Yet even patients with critical ischaemia may continue to smoke. But that is another story!

Yours sincerely

FOOT CARE:
ADVICE FOR PATIENTS

- Wear well-fitting, round-toed shoes
- Wear woollen socks to keep the feet warm
- Examine both feet and shoes (for foreign objects) daily
- Keep feet clean by daily washing, then dry thoroughly
- Use moisturising creams for dry skin
- Cut nails along the contours of the toes
- Corns and calluses should not be treated except by a State Registered Podiatrist

COMMANDMENT

Take immediate action in cases of infected tissue around a foot ulcer

The colour, general condition and appearance of the foot must be noted. Any abnormality of the nails, or the presence of corns or calluses, allows one to refer to the podiatrist while indicating forcibly that these are conditions which should not be treated by amateurs. Skin breaks, ulcers and bony deformities merit aggressive therapy.

COMMANDMENT
Tell smokers that their feet are at risk

MANAGEMENT OF THE DIABETIC FOOT

The management of established foot disease takes second place to its prevention and the concept of screening is not appropriate here. However, much can be done to improve established disease.

Neuropathy

Painful neuropathy may be exacerbated by alcohol and drugs such as metronidazole. The standard treatment for the pain is a tricyclic antidepressant, which helps in over 50% of cases. Start with a small dose of amitriptyline, say 10–25 mg at night, and increase slowly up to 75 mg. Carbamazepine and mexiletine have also been tried, but are probably not effective. A bed-cradle may diminish nocturnal hyperaesthesia.

Painless neuropathy is managed by obsessional attention to foot care. Involving a relative may be helpful.

COMMANDMENT
Remember that painful neuropathy is treatable

Dr AJC Pickering,
The Village Surgery

Dear Charles

I would value your help with Robert Wesley, a jolly 68 year old who has Type II diabetes quite well controlled on insulin. His wife is a most capable former nurse. The immediate problem is of claudication, starting after about 150 yards and relieved by rest. The picture, however, is muddled by his marked shortness of breath. I could detect no pulses in either leg though his microcirculation, as evidenced by foot temperature and return of skin colour after compression, seems good. He does not suffer from night pain. He has diminished vibration sense, though his reflexes are normal, and is overweight at 114 kg for a height of 1.74 m. His alcohol intake is modest now, though I imagine it may have been substantial in the past as he was in the Navy.

Robert has a large heart on chest X-ray though I could detect no abnormal sounds in the chest and his JVP is not visible. The ECG shows some lateral ischaemia. Renal function is OK as assessed by a normal creatinine.

Is Robert's problem vascular disease alone, vascular disease and modest heart failure, or a combination of both of these and obesity? He complains of restricted mobility through pain. Should we be thinking of investigating his vasculature with a view to reconstructive surgery, or is the easier option to treat his apparently mild heart failure? I don't think modification of his weight is realistic.

I would, as ever, value your advice.

Yours sincerely

Tony

**Dr Charles Fox, The Diabetes Centre,
District General Hospital**

Dear Tony
Thank you for your letter about Robert Wesley. I would list his medical problems as follows:

- Peripheral vascular disease (severe but not critical)
- Neuropathy (asymptomatic)
- Cardiac failure, ?hypertensive
- Obesity, BMI 38

People with peripheral vascular disease often seem to soldier on for years in a fairly stable condition. However, one should never become complacent because there is always a risk of something triggering a sudden deterioration. Such triggers include injury from new shoes, infection from careless home podiatry or, more commonly, cardiac failure – in which the fall in cardiac output reduces the already precarious peripheral blood supply. Oedema of the feet may be a further adverse factor by compressing the thready arterioles. I would suggest the following management plan:

1. First, treat Robert's cardiac failure with an ACE inhibitor, which will not cause dehydration.
2. Then treat his peripheral vascular disease. Since you cannot find any pulses in his legs, he probably has large vessel disease. This means he is a candidate for reconstructive surgery or angioplasty. Unfortunately, most surgeons hesitate to perform elective surgery when the risks are increased by obesity. Angioplasty is also technically difficult in overweight patient. This is due to the difficulty in angling the needle used in arterial puncture down the femoral artery. The catheter used in arteriograms is inserted cephalically, against the flow of blood, but the angioplasty catheter has to be directed towards the distal block.
3. I agree Robert is not going to change his weight, but it is a major obstacle to successful relief of his claudication.
   Yours sincerely

Arthropathy

Neuropathic arthropathy was described by Jean-Martin Charcot, in 1868. Charcot changes are not uncommon in a neuropathic diabetic foot. The process is heralded by pain, often following a trivial injury. The mid-tarsal joint becomes hot and swollen. The process usually progresses remorselessly until the foot is permanently deformed with a high risk of future ulceration. This problem should be referred urgently as there is some evidence that early treatment with pamidronate can halt the process.

The severely painful foot

Firstly, decide whether the likely problem is neuropathy or ischaemia.

Painful neuropathy

This is treated as described, using a tricyclic antidepressant. The hospital pain clinic may be able to help – for instance, by supplying a TENS machine.

Amyotrophy

Amyotrophy is a rare condition causing severe intractable pain, usually in one leg and and ALWAYS associated with extreme weight loss. Despite the severity of the pain, the patient can be reassured with confidence that the pain will ease after a period of six to twelve months and, in time, clear up completely.

Ischaemia

This is a more likely explanation if only one foot is involved. The foot will be cold and pulseless, with discoloration progressing from that of pre-gangrene (a brick-red flush in a painful ischaemic foot), through little black tips to some of the toes, to the large black patches of frank gangrene. Vasodilators are not effective, but beta blockers may cause further vasoconstriction and should be discontinued. If the pain persists, the site of arterial stenosis should be identified by angiography or Duplex Doppler with a view to angioplasty or bypass surgery.

COMMANDMENT

Be prepared to prescribe opiates for ischaemic pain

If the addicted patient finds giving up smoking difficult, weight loss is, in practice, well nigh impossible. Badgering the obese to lose weight, implying that they are weak or blame-worthy, serves if anything to reinforce whichever psychological mechanisms have contributed to overeating in the first place. Gentle and respectful encouragement, with praise for effort and jubilation at success, may be more effective and certainly less stressful for both patient and health professional.

Ulcers

As usual, the first rule in diabetic foot disease is to decide whether the ulcer is caused by ischaemia, neuropathy or both (see Figure 11.1). The decision can usually be made on clinical grounds. It is also important to decide whether the ulcer is infected.

Figure 11.1

Pointers to neuropathic / ischaemic ulcers

	Neuropathic	Ischaemic
Appearance	Swollen	Wasted
	Red/normal	Black/red
	Deformed foot	Normal shaped foot
Pain	None or mild	Severe
Temperature	Warm	Cold
Pulses	Present	Absent
Sensation	Absent	Very sensitive
Callus	Present	Absent
Prognosis	Reasonable	Poor

Neuropathic ulcer without infection

This is serious, but not usually an emergency. Refer for urgent podiatric opinion. The podiatrist will remove any callus and, if healing is delayed, will make a customised cast with a window cut over the ulcer. This allows healing while preserving mobility. Many patients need encouragement actually to wear a cast. We have an old friend with a longstanding neuropathic ulcer who brings his cast along to the clinic in a plastic bag "just in case he needs it".

Neuropathic ulcer with infection

A small area of cellulitis around an ulcer need not cause panic provided urgent podiatry referral can be arranged. Take a swab and start treatment with co-amoxiclav while awaiting sensitivities. However, if the foot is generally warm and there is any suspicion of deep seated infection, arrange urgent admission. Immediate treatment will include intravenous antibiotics, thorough debridement by the surgeon or podiatrist, daily dressings and inspection, and avoidance of weight-bearing.

Figure 11.2

Antibiotic choices in diabetic foot infections

NB: TAKE SWAB BEFORE STARTING ANTIBIOTICS

■ Topical antibiotics have NO place in diabetic foot ulcers

■ While awaiting results, start co-amoxiclav

■ Add metronidazole in severe infections

■ In osteomyelitis, try clindamycin or ciprofloxacin

Once the infection starts to improve, antibiotics can be given by mouth, but exhaustive debridement must be continued regularly since the infection may be deep seated.

If the ulcer fails to heal, there may be underlying osteomyelitis which is commonly seen in diabetic feet with severe neuropathic damage. X-ray appearances may look alarming, but bony infection in diabetes can be relatively benign and may even be cured by antibiotics. Clindamycin and ciprofloxacin have high bone penetration and are particularly effective. Simple X-rays do not disclose whether the infection is active. MRI scanning reliably detects active infection and has taken the guesswork out of managing chronic osteo-myelitis in diabetic feet.

Ischaemic ulcer

These are usually very painful, requiring slow release morphine for relief. In the frail elderly, the combination of severe pain and morphine may lead to mental confusion which makes nursing difficult.

In a severe ischaemic ulcer, amputation may be inevitable, but before this irrevocable step, the vascular supply must be assessed to ensure that no reconstructive procedure is possible. Angiography is the standard procedure but Duplex Doppler can provide a non-invasive but quantitative evaluation of limb blood flow. Either method will reveal lesions treatable by angioplasty or a bypass operation. Reconstructive surgical technique continues to improve, and the distal end of a graft can now be attached to foot arteries, with good results.

Amputation

This is the stark end-point of diabetic foot care.

In some cases, the decision to amputate is clear. In a patient with severe pain from extensive gangrene, the only humane course of action is major amputation. If the patient is not confused, it is important to talk him or her through the procedure. Suffering intractable pain, many patients are only too keen to have the source of their agony removed. Amputation usually provides dramatic relief, though phantom pain may be a problem, especially if the pain has been longstanding.

Many patients, however, have a mixed picture with neuropathy, infection and necrosis. If the pain is under control and not keeping them awake, it is best to explain to the patient that amputation is a possibility and wait for the reaction. Some people are completely devastated by the thought of losing a leg while others remain stoical. Try to involve the patient in the decision, and be prepared to bide your time if the patient is psychologically unready. Amputation forced onto a reluctant patient may appear cost-effective by reducing length of stay but, in the long term, it can lead to excess morbidity and prolonged rehabilitation.

NEUROPATHY 12

Neuropathy is the hidden complication of diabetes, but amongst the diabetic population it probably causes the greatest amount of discomfort and distress. Blindness, amputation and renal failure are the three great threats which menace everyone with this disease, but there are strategies for dealing with these high-profile dangers. Thus we screen for retinopathy and nephropathy and run "foot at risk" clinics. The latter deal in part with neuropathy, but nerve damage affects parts of the body that other complications do not reach. Many diabetic complications are related to the degree of metabolic control, but some of the most painful and distressing neuropathic complications discussed in this section may affect patients with exemplary control.

Neuropathy has its most obvious manifestation in the problems affecting the lower limbs. The nerves which supply the toes have their origin and cell nucleus over a metre away in the lumbar spine. Thus any pathological process causing damage to nerves is likely to harm those vulnerable structures. The main threat to the diabetic foot is peripheral vascular disease, which may be amplified by the presence of neuropathy (see Chapter 11).

Diabetic neuropathy is always divided into peripheral and autonomic types. This classification is of value in grouping together likely associations, but in practice most neuropathic complications present as a ragbag of isolated complaints.

We shall stick to the traditional grouping but will highlight those problems which are particularly prevalent or devastating to the patient.

As feet have been covered in the previous chapter, this one will deal mainly with neuropathy outside the foot.

PERIPHERAL NEUROPATHY

The mechanism of nerve damage is not well understood. There are two main hypotheses. The first proposes the accumulation within the nerve of sorbitol derived from the excess serum glucose. This interferes with nerve conduction, possibly by causing the nerve to swell. A group of drugs, aldose reductase inhibitors, were developed at great expense in the hope that reducing the concentration of sorbitol would allow the nerves to regain their normal function. Sadly this endeavour seems to have failed, although aldose reductase inhibitors still have their proponents.

Other drugs which may help neuropathic symptoms are undergoing clinical trials. Acetyl carnitine looks promising in animal studies, and initial work with diabetic patients suggests that it improves nerve conduction and reduces painful symptoms. This needs to be confirmed in formal double blind studies.

An alternative hypothesis holds that diabetic neuropathy results from damage to small blood vessels which actually supply nutrients to the nerves. This puts it in the same category as retinopathy and nephropathy. By taking serial biopsies of peripheral nerve in the leg, research workers have obtained dramatic pictures showing destruction of the small arteries which accompany the nerve bundles. Neither of these hypotheses has been developed into a unifying theory of the causation of diabetic nerve disease.

Carpal tunnel syndrome

This is a common neurological diagnosis associated with a number of conditions, including diabetes. The median nerve passes through the wrist in a small bony canal and is kept in place by a strap of ligament called the flexor retinaculum. If the nerve swells, it is compressed by the surrounding structures, a condition described as entrapment neuropathy. The median nerve supplies skin sensation on the palmar side of the hand over the thumb and index, middle and ring fingers. It also supplies muscles at the base of the thumb and the ulnar side of the hand (the thenar and hypothenar eminences).

COMMANDMENT

Consider the possibility of myxoedema in a patient, especially with diabetes, who presents with carpal tunnel syndrome

The diagnosis of carpal tunnel syndrome can usually be made from the history. It first causes painful "pins and needles" in the fingers, which often wakes the patient at night, and is relieved by shaking the hand about. During the day, the pain, which may radiate back up the forearm, is usually precipitated by wrist movements (e.g. wringing out washing) and is helped by resting. The diagnosis should be confirmed by clinical examination and simple nerve function studies (EMG) specifically to confirm a compression neuropathy. If there is significant slowing of nerve conduction at the level of the wrist, it is worth suggesting a decompression operation if measures such as steroid injections are ineffective. This can be done as a day case and often gives several years' relief.

If any patient presents with symptoms of carpal tunnel syndrome, it is important to think of other causes such as myxoedema, acromegaly and pregnancy. It also occurs in patients with damage to the wrist bones, as in rheumatoid arthritis.

Other entrapment neuropathies

Carpel tunnel is by far the most common example of a nerve suffering compression. Other examples in diabetes are the ulnar nerve, which may become injured at the elbow, causing pain over the little finger and border of the hand, leading on to a characteristic claw hand deformity. Ulnar nerve entrapment needs urgent referral; the ulnar nerve is not forgiving.

The common peroneal nerve may be damaged as it winds round the neck of the fibula. This may lead to the rare complication of foot drop.

Painful diabetic amyotrophy

This is not a common problem but because of its remarkable natural history, the few cases seen make quite an impression. The story usually starts with a NIDD, either newly diagnosed or with reasonable control on tablets, who over the course of a few days develops severe pain and wasting in one of the thighs. Apart from the dramatic wasting of the quadriceps, there may not be much else to find on examination. However, the patient complains bitterly of unremitting pain which often has an affect on appetite, causing generalised weight loss. In even more unusual cases, the pain and weakness may affect the abdominal wall so that intra-abdominal pathology is suspected.

Some authorities believe that this condition may be improved by tight control, usually with insulin. However, it seems that given time the problem rights itself whatever the state of the blood sugar. Unfortunately the process of recovery takes up to two years, by which time the patient will have had a large number of unhelpful neurological investigations, and faith in his medical advisors will be wearing pretty thin.

Ophthalmoplegia

Unlike painful amyotrophy, ophthalmoplegia is relatively common in diabetes. It is sometimes painful at the onset and always recovers completely within one to nine months, i.e. more rapidly than amyotrophy. For more details, see the section on diabetic eye disease in Chapter 10.

Cheiroarthropathy

This is a common finding in young people with diabetes and has been the subject of many research projects. It results in fixed flexion of the finger joints so that the fingers cannot be fully extended. This can be demonstrated by the so-called "prayer sign" where the patient is unable to put the palms of the hands flat together. It is thought to be neuropathic in origin, and is more common in young people with poorly-controlled diabetes dating from childhood.

AUTONOMIC NEUROPATHY

By definition none of us is aware of our autonomic nervous system, which quietly looks after our wellbeing. Only when it starts to fail do we become aware of its importance and how difficult it is to put it right. Diabetes is the most common cause of autonomic nerve failure. We have seen that diabetic damage to peripheral nerves may present with isolated symptoms. On the other hand, if one system is affected by autonomic neuropathy, there is a good chance that abnormalities can be detected in other systems, often at a subclinical level.

Impotence

Finding out about the problem

Dealing well with impotence takes a lot of time – not a plentiful commodity in the National Health Service. It is important to take a full history, finding out what the patient sees as the problem, and while asking about drugs, alcohol and smoking. The partner's attitude to the problem is a vital part of the assessment and may influence the outcome of any treatment that is tried. Finally ask the patient what he expects in the way of treatment.

Nomenclature

The term "impotence" is now politically incorrect. It implies that simply because of a problem with sex, a man loses all his power. "Erectile failure" or "erectile insufficiency" are suitable alternatives. We will stick with the familiar term in this edition but it may help when talking to patients to refer to the "difficulty they have getting an erection" rather than the expression "impotence" which has a stark and hopeless ring to it.

Prevalence

The prevalence of impotence in the diabetic male population has been much argued about. There have been disputes about the frequency of impotence in the "normal" population and whether it really is more common in diabetes. Some believe that a chronic illness with a reputation for causing impotence would be enough to stop most men in their tracks, and that impotence in diabetic men is mainly caused by psychological factors.

Whatever the cause there are many men with diabetes (approximately 30% in the average hospital clinic) whose lives are made miserable by their inability to lead a normal sex life. This may lead to marital breakdown – a heavy price to pay for having diabetes. The problem of impotence is equally prevalent in patients seen in GP clinics.

In older men with diabetes, impotence does not seem to be related to the degree of metabolic control.

Possible causes of erectile failure in diabetic men

It may be difficult to pinpoint the exact cause in many patients. However, we need to understand the possible mechanisms so that we can discuss the various treatment options with our patients. In simple terms, achieving an erection requires an intact neurological system, an adequate supply of blood, the correct balance of sex hormones and a brain which can initiate the process rather than blocking it. In considering the history it is important to establish whether spontaneous erections occur, for example on waking.

1. Autonomic neuropathy

This is the most common cause of impotence in diabetic men. The diagnosis is simple if there are signs of neuropathy affecting other systems. In some cases the rest of the nervous system seems to be intact and the diagnosis is made by exclusion.

2. Vascular insufficiency

Once again this problem may be obvious, from a history of claudication and the absence of peripheral pulses. If there is any doubt, non-invasive blood flow studies may provide useful information and indicate the need for arteriography. Some centres are using Doppler ultrasound to assess the blood pressure in the penile artery. Patients who smoke need reminding that smoking damages arteries.

3.   Hormonal abnormalities

In a full assessment of a patient with impotence, it is important to rule out endocrine causes such as a low serum testosterone level, or a raised serum prolactin level.

4.   Drugs

Antihypertensive drugs (including thiazide diuretics and beta blockers) may cause impotence. A drug holiday may cheer up a patient immensely. Psychotropic drugs may also lead to impotence.

5.   Alcohol

Some patients are surprised to discover that alcohol may reduce the capacity to get an erection without reducing the libido.

6.   Psychological factors

These are likely to play a part in diabetic impotence when reduced self-esteem exacerbates the problem. Suspect a psychological cause when impotence has developed suddenly and when it is not absolute.

Treatment of erectile failure

Talking

This is the most important part of the treatment. The patient needs detailed explanation, and discussions about treatment options. Ideally the partner should be present as a successful result will depend on her support.

Tablets

These may be a help to patients with a primary psychological cause. Yohimbine is recommended by some experts.

Vacuum devices

These work by engorging the penis with blood to give an erection which is maintained by a rubber ring at the base of the penis. The devices are expensive (around £100) and have a satisfaction rate of 60–80%.

Intracavernosal injections

Undoubtedly, these can be effective and we have several patients who regularly ask for a prescription for papaverine to be injected into the side of the penis. This is clearly a viable option for some people. The injections may cause fibrosis and there is a small risk of priapism which would have to be decompressed surgically. Recently prostaglandin E1 (Alprostadil) has been found to be as effective, with less risk of scarring from repeated injections.

Surgery

A last resort is surgically to insert a semi-rigid rod into the corpus cavernosum. Some patients are very pleased with the results.

In an ideal world, diabetic men with this distressing condition would receive integrated care from a diabetologist, a specialist in psychosexual disorders, and a urologist. At present there are very few centres able to provide this. Meanwhile, an interested GP and practice nurse can supply a better service than is available in many hospitals.

A useful patient information leaflet, written by Dr Bill Alexander, is available from Owen Mumford (see Appendix 3).

Gastrointestinal problems

After impotence, these are probably the autonomic complications which cause most distress. They are caused by degeneration of the nerve supply to the gut, with or without bacterial overgrowth.

Gastric stasis

This can cause vomiting and regurgitation of food. Pressure studies may show failure of normal motor cycles in the stomach with pyloric spasm. Metoclopramide, domperidone or cisapride may promote gastric emptying. Erythromycin has been shown to be effective and should be tried

Diarrhoea

In most cases this is an inconvenience which at worst causes an embarrassing incident while the patient is out and about. At the other end of the spectrum are rare cases where life is ruined by frequent episodes of severe explosive diarrhoea. If there is accompanying lack of anal tone the patient may have to live with the constant risk of faecal incontinence, which is often nocturnal.

The first line of treatment is codeine phosphate or Lomotil. Sometimes metoclopramide can help.

The next step is to try oxytetracycline 250 mg tds. If this works at all, it usually does so after the first few doses, presumably by correcting bacterial overgrowth.

It is difficult to assess the efficacy of treatment for a problem which is intermittent and prone to spontaneous remissions. In refractory cases, some patients are helped by Creon although there is no convincing evidence for exocrine pancreatic damage as a cause of diabetic diarrhoea. Some centres claim sporadic success with cholestyramine.

Cardiovascular problems

Loss of cardiovascular reflexes in diabetes has been the source of countless research projects, but causes little in the way of symptoms. These include loss of beat to beat variation, abnormal Valsalva response and minor reduction in blood pressure on standing. In rare cases, postural hypotension can be a serious problem. This usually occurs in people with other evidence of autonomic damage and serves to make their lives even more wretched. In such cases it is vital to ensure that the patient is not taking any drugs which might excerbate the problem. If hypotension is causing troublesome symptoms, any antihypertensive treatment has to be reduced. Other possible culprits are diuretics and antidepressants. Active treatment includes encouraging fluid retention, in the hope of increasing the standing blood pressure. Non steroidal anti-inflammatory drugs have a mild fluid-retaining effect, and patients may also be helped by fludrocortisone. Start with 100 μg daily and increase to a maximum of 400 μg. Obviously, successful fluid retention risks provoking cardiac failure.

Dr AJC Pickering,
The Village Surgery

Dear Charles

Would you advise me on whether to investigate people with diabetes who develop diarrhoea.

I am thinking about a 52 year old train driver, Cecil Newsome, who has had diabetes for five years and has since taken metformin 500 mg twice daily. He was overweight at the time of diagnosis (BMI 32) and has not been able to lose weight.

For the past month, Cecil has been passing soft faeces with some urgency, four or five times a day. He has not noticed blood or mucus in the faeces. His weight is steady. There is no orthostatic hypotension or evidence of neuropathy elsewhere. As you might imagine, this bowel habit is not easily accommodated in his work. Accordingly, we have prescribed codeine phosphate.

Can I assume this symptom is a side-effect of the metformin or evidence of autonomic neuropathy, or should I organise investigations to exclude bowel cancer or inflammatory bowel disease? I do not wish to cause alarm by suggesting investigations but I would not like to delay investigations by, for example, a trial of a different oral hypoglycaemic.

Can I assume that after five years, diarrhoea would not suddenly become a side-effect of metformin? Does autonomic neuropathy of the bowel occur in isolation and so suddenly? Should we adopt a policy of investigating all such cases, the penalty of missing treatable bowel cancer being so severe?

Yours sincerely

Tony

Postural hypotension is caused by a deficiency of venous return, leading to relative hypovolaemia. Firm support stockings may provide some relief.

It is important to remember that myocardial infarction is more likely to be painless in people with diabetes, presumably due to degeneration of mediastinal pain fibres.

Dr Charles Fox, The Diabetes Centre,
District General Hospital

Dear Tony
    Thank you for asking me about Cecil and the
problem of frequent bowel actions which must make train driving difficult.
The likely culprit is indeed metformin and there is often a delay between the
start of treatment and onset of gastrointestinal side-effects. Since he is only
taking 500 mg twice daily, a dose reduction is not likely to help. Stopping
metformin should cause a rapid improvement in the diarrhoea, though Cecil
is likely to need a sulphonylurea as an alternative to control his blood
glucose. Gliclazide would be a resonable choice – the side-effects being
hypoglycaemia and an increase in body weight.
    If I am wrong and he continues to suffer with diarrhoea after stop-
ping metformin, you will have to look for other causes. Many patients suffer
with diabetic diarrhoea but they are usually IDDs with other manifestations
of autonomic neuropathy such as delayed gastric emptying and bladder
disturbance. Cecil does not fall into this category and I agree that you
should play safe and rule out bowel cancer by barium enema or
colonoscopy.
    Yours sincerely

Genito-urinary problems

Bladder disturbances

These are common in diabetes but fortunately they are usually
subclinical, and many patients are unaware that they have a
large floppy bladder. At a later stage of disease, the patient
will notice a poor stream and overflow incontinence. Uro-
dynamic investigations will rule out a treatable cause, such
as prostatic enlargement. Drug therapy with cholinergic agents
is disappointing and patients with these problems are best
served by mechanical methods – such as simple manual

pressure or even intermittent self-catheterisation. Prophylactic antibiotics are justified in people with recurrent urinary infections.

Retrograde ejaculation

This is another consequence of autonomic failure but, unlike impotence, is only a serious problem if the man is wanting to have children.

Sweating disturbances

Lack of sweating, causing dry skin, may be a factor in diabetic foot problems. However, it is not normally noticeable unless there is a compensatory increase in sweating of the trunk and upper limbs.

Gustatory sweating is a rare but well-known symptom whereby, immediately after eating food, there is profuse sweating of the face and head. This may be unilateral which suggests that it results from aberrant regeneration of autonomic nerves.

Pupillary reflexes

Pupillary reflexes have been studied extensively in diabetes and, although abnormalities are a quantifiable marker of autonomic neuropathy, they do not lead to any symptoms and their detection will probably remain a research tool.

NEPHROPATHY 13

There is an awful sense of fatalism about renal failure in diabetes, though it is not a particularly common complication. Pirart, in his outstanding study of the natural history of diabetes, found that only 14% of 4400 patients studied for up to 25 years developed nephropathy.

However, once proteinuria is detected, the patient seems to take a steady downward path. This may end either in end-stage renal failure (ESRF) or more commonly in premature death from cardiovascular disease.

Most patients find out sooner rather than later that they have a disease which threatens their kidneys. This is a difficult threat to contemplate, partly because the person in the street (and for that matter the average doctor) cannot really visualise the necessity of being hooked up to a machine three times a week. It is horrible to contemplate blindness or losing a leg, but at least this is something with which everyone can identify.

While nephropathy remains a real fear in diabetes, there have been some advances in the past few years which help us to be look on it more positively.

RISK FACTORS AND ASSOCIATED COMPLICATIONS

Because of the way the results are presented in the DCCT (see Chapter 3), it is difficult to extract data about the development of complications. However, in the group with tight control, the risk of proteinuria is reduced by 39%.

The UKPDS (also discussed in Chapter 3) is a multicentre study of people with NIDDM. Results to date suggest that 4% of patients have Albustix-positive albuminuria. Microalbuminuria (the earliest sign of kidney damage) was much more common in those patients with hypertension (24%) than those with normal blood pressure (14%). This striking association of hypertension with other risk factors is considered in more detail in Chapter 14.

PERCEPTIONS OF RENAL DISEASE

Diabetic renal disease can be divided into five stages. Patients will, of course, have different perceptions of their problems depending on the stage they may have reached. In order to help them come to terms with their situation, it is worth trying to consider how the patient is thinking. Finding out the perceptions of the patient is the first step in education.

Stage 1: No detectable abnormality

At this stage, patients must know why they are asked to bring a urine sample to each annual review (i.e. proteinuria is much more significant than glycosuria). If a screening programme for microalbuminuria (MA) is in place, the details of the procedure must be explained to the patient, and the implications of a positive test discussed. The patient should be given the opportunity to opt out of testing for MA, but given that MA represents a reversible stage in the process, most patients are keen to be tested.

Stage 2:   Microalbuminuria

If the patient has been properly prepared for a positive test, he or she should be prepared to take an ACE inhibitor and to work to improve diabetic control. A number of patients will find it no easier to achieve tight control once they know that they have kidney disease than they did before there was any evidence of such complications. At this and all stages of diabetes, it is dangerous to attach any blame to patients for their failure to "come up to scratch". People are more likely to adopt a policy of changing for the better if they feel "good" about themselves. Self-care follows self-esteem. In most cases, diabetes remains a disease which is difficult to control and professionals must avoid minimising the problems faced by their patients.

Stage 3:   Proteinuria

The key elements to this stage are effective blood pressure control and regular creatinine measurements to detect the early loss of renal function. This stage may last from six to 15 years and allows plenty of time for the patient to come to terms with the prospect of renal replacement therapy.

Stage 4:   Chronic renal failure

The process of remorseless increase in serum creatinine is often compounded by other diabetic problems such as pro- liferative retinopathy or foot ulcers. It is important to listen carefully for such symptoms as angina and claudication and to be on the look out for problems in the eyes and feet. With each new manifestation of large and small vessel disease, the patient may feel increasingly under attack from the disease.

Stage 5:   End stage renal failure

The few patients who reach this stage often feel a sense of relief (akin to the sense of accomplishment that patients often feel after starting insulin). In fact there are many parallels between starting dialysis and starting insulin. In both cases, there is the problem of learning the technical side of the disease together with all the jargon at a time when the patient and relatives are trying to cope with the emotional shock of a serious medical problem. The difference, however, is that only 50% of patients in this group live for more than three years on dialysis.

PROTEINURIA

This is the standard way of defining diabetic renal damage at an early stage. Put like that, proteinuria does not sound particularly serious but, after 40 years of diabetes, only 10% of patients with proteinuria survive in contrast to 70% of those without. Once proteinuria has appeared, there is a steady decline towards end stage renal failure. The rate of decline varies from one patient to another but averages out at about ten years. Because it appears to be a mundane and innocuous procedure, patients may underestimate the significance of the detection of proteinuria.

A spot urine sample is tested using a dipstick such as Albustix (Bayer Diagnostics) and this simple and reliable test should be incorporated into the annual review. Avoid a sample that may be contaminated by blood during menstruation. If the result is negative the patient should be told the good news and asked to supply another sample at the next annual review. A trace of proteinuria can simply be noted though it is probably worth taking the time to explain that it is partic-ularly important to repeat the test in 12 months. If unequivocal proteinuria is detected for the first time, it is worth arranging urine culture to rule out a symptomless urinary infection. The presence of proteinuria should trigger a blood test to measure serum creatinine.

TEACHING POINT

If a patient is found to have proteinuria, effective control of blood pressure will slow progression of renal damage

What action should be taken?

It should be a reflex action to take the blood pressure once proteinuria has been detected in a patient with diabetes. If the reading is greater than 140/90, aim to reduce the blood pressure at to 130/85.

The majority of diabetic patients who develop proteinuria have diabetic nephropathy and therefore do not need a renal biopsy to establish the diagnosis. However, in rare cases where there is could be an alternative explanation (such as an autoimmune disease), a biopsy may be necessary.

MICROALBUMINURIA (MA)

This is defined as a measurable urinary protein excretion which is below the level detected by Albustix. Between 10 and 15%

Dr AJC Pickering,
The Village Surgery

Dear Charles
    What advice would you offer about screening for microalbuminuria?
    At the moment, we test the urine for albumin in all those who attend our diabetic clinic. I believe, however, that microalbuminuria is a sensitive marker for deterioration in renal function in IDDM, so should we systematically test this group? If so with what frequency? If there is an association between nephropathy and other forms of microvascular disease, might we further define the population at risk by focusing our attention (and indeed the resources of our beleaguered NHS) on, for example, IDDs with retinopathy or hypertension? As I understand it, the latter are at particular risk of nephropathy.
    What about NIDDM and screening for microalbuminuria? I understand there is no evidence for suggesting that this type of screening is helpful, but is there any logic to favour it?
    On the wider subject of renal function, I continue to be confused by the co-existence of a change in "normal" serum creatinine levels with age and rising serum creatinine in nephropathy. Given a slightly elevated creatinine level in a NIDDM, do I take this to be "normal" for age or the sign of early renal failure? Would creatinine clearance tests help? Or is the serum creatinine as sensitive an indicator as the clearance?
    Yours aye

    Tony

of IDDs will have MA on repeated testing. Such patients carry a twentyfold risk of developing renal failure compared with IDDs who do not have MA. This alarming situation is to some extent softened by the fact that MA is a reversible stage of renal disease. By tightening up metabolic control and treatment with an ACE inhibitor, MA can be abolished in many patients.

MA is also a risk factor in NIDDM, but it is associated more strongly with cardiovascular disease than with renal failure. So far it has not been shown that in NIDDM, MA can be

**Dr Charles Fox, The Diabetes Centre,
District General Hospital**

Dear Tony

Microalbuminuria (MA) is a indicator of early renal damage at a stage when it may be reversible. True albuminuria (detectable with a dipstick) is a marker of irreversible nephropathy and sooner or later the serum creatinine will inexorably climb to the level of end-stage renal failure (ESRF) with the need for dialysis or transplant.

MA cannot simply be measured like any other test. It is important to explain in advance that a positive test is Bad News and puts the patient in a higher risk category for developing kidney failure or heart disease. The Good News is that these risks can be reduced by improving diabetic control and taking a tablet that will protect their kidneys.

It takes time to organise a microalbuminuria screening service and there some important questions to be considered:

1. Should we go to the trouble of measuring MA?
Some experts maintain that since all patients should aim at tight metabolic and BP control, the presence or absence of MA should not alter our management. The contrary view is that tight blood glucose control increases the risk of hypoglycaemia which has its own morbidity and mortality. There is also the ethical point that if someone is at increased risk, they have the right to know – provided they want to be told.

2. What urine sample should we use for measuring MA?
In the General Hospital, we have decided on three early morning samples for measuring the albumin/creatinine ratio. If these are above the threshold, and urinary infection has been ruled out, the patient will be defined as microalbuminuria positive.

3. On whom and how frequently should we measure MA?
Start screening IDDs, irrespective of age. MA is associated with cardiovascular events in NIDDM, as it is in people who do not have diabetes. However, MA represents renal damage at a reversible stage and the evidence for this reversibility is much stronger in IDDM than in NIDDM.

4. How should we educate patients before we measure MA?
The presence of MA in a patient with IDDM increases by twentyfold the risk of developing nephropathy and carries a greatly increased risk of cardiovascular disease. Because of the implications of a positive test, we must give patients enough information to allow them to decide whether or not they want to be tested and to realise that a positive test will put them under pressure. We must be prepared to help them deal with emotional and medical anxieties arising from the test.

5. What should we tell patients if they are MA positive?

If we have kept them fully informed about the implications of having MA, patients should understand the need to improve their blood glucose control and to keep their blood pressure normal. Patients react to news in different ways — some will be positive, others fatalistic. It is up to us to harness their energies as best we can.

6. How would we change our management of patients with MA?

Ideally, all patients should strive to maintain immaculate metabolic control in order to reduce the risk of complications. However, in the real world, any added risk may provide the incentive to take diabetes more seriously. The message is:

Aim for near-perfect diabetic control
Keep blood pressure near-normal
Stop smoking

Thus there are both logistic and educational problems in the introduction of MA screening.

If MA is the beginning of the story, the beginning of the final chapter is a rising serum creatinine. At normal levels, creatinine measurements have a poor reproducibility (about ±10%) but the results become more accurate as the level rises above normal. The kidney is almost entirely responsible for excreting creatinine, the production of which is influenced by such factors as overall muscle mass, dietary protein intake and age. Creatinine clearance estimations rely on accurate saving of all the urine produced in a 24 hour period, and can themselves be inaccurate. The trend in serial creatinine measurements is what matters and I would simply repeat the test in three or four months.

Yours sincerely

reversed by improving control or giving ACE inhibitors. For this reason, the main thrust of using MA as an early warning system for future trouble has been directed at IDDM.

Problems with MA

It must seem that every diabetes centre should act quickly to set up a foolproof plan for MA screening, so that patients who are positive can take steps to improve their chances of remaining healthy. Unfortunately there are problems which have to be solved before MA screening can be introduced:

1. Education of patients and their relatives
2. Cost (in relation to prevalence)
3. Which system and what threshold
4. Organisation (including training of staff)

There are different ways of expressing microalbuminuria, which further confuses all but the experts. Since we have to use hard numbers, Figure 13.1 is included to help comparison:

The test requires a 24 hour urine collection to measure 24 hour albumin excretion. This may work in a research laboratory, but is impractical for a routine clinic in a district general hospital where MA is being used as a screening test for nephropathy. The creatinine concentration of the urine

Figure 13.1

Different ways of expressing microalbuminuria

Normal	<20 mg min^{-1}	<30 mg day^{-1}
Microalbuminuria	20–200 mg min^{-1}	30–300 mg day^{-1}
Albuminuria	200 mg min^{-1}	>300 mg day^{-1}

NB: albumin/creatinine ratio greater than 3.5 predicts an albumin excretion rate of 30 mg/min

is an approximate indicator of urine flow rate, so an albumin/creatinine ratio measurement on a spot urine specimen avoids the need for a timed sample. Apart from glomerular damage, the albumin excretion rate may be increased by exercise, by urinary infection or by contamination during menstruation. It is lowest when the subject is lying down and the preferred urine specimen is that passed immediately on rising.

The threshold for microalbuminuria varies from 2–3.5 mg/mmol and each diabetic centre will have to decide where to pitch its cut-off for calling a particular value "microalbuminuria positive". This will depend on how sensitive the centre's staff want to make their system.

Prevalence

In a population of IDDs under the age of 70 years, between 10 and 15% of patients will have established microalbuminuria. The range for NIDDs is quoted as 8–46%, but as it is not known to be a reversible risk factor in NIDDM, screening is usually offered first to IDDs.

ESTABLISHED RENAL FAILURE

Patients with proteinuria and a raised creatinine need special treatment. Measure the serum creatinine every six months, to assess the rate of decline of renal function. Tight control of blood pressure and blood glucose will protect the kidneys, though for patients on insulin it may be more difficult than usual to achieve smooth glycaemic control. This is probably because insulin is partly metabolised by the kidneys and its duration of action is thus more variable than usual. Patients in renal failure usually need to reduce their total insulin dose to avoid hypos.

Approximately 30% of patients in renal failure will be NIDDs and provided their metabolic control is reasonable, they can

IMPORTANT POINTS

■ Once serum creatinine rises above normal, test every six months – more frequently if there is a sudden jump in values.

■ Creatinine clearance is a better measure of renal function, but is tedious for patients and is completely inaccurate if the urine collection is incomplete.

■ Once serum creatinine reaches 150 μmol/l, only 50% of renal function remains.

■ A low protein diet certainly slows down deterioration in renal function, but it is irksome for patients who are already restricting fats and simple carbohydrates. It increases the risk of patients becoming malnourished.

■ Remember to check serum calcium in patients with chronic renal failure. If it starts to fall below normal, consider prescribing vitamin D in the form of "One Alpha".

■ During this phase of worsening renal failure, screen carefully for other complications, in particular hypertension, retinopathy, angina and peripheral vascular disease.

■ Heavy proteinuria (>3.5 g/24 hrs) leading to nephrotic syndrome is rare but difficult to treat and may need in-patient care.

■ If there is no joint Diabetic Renal Clinic, patients with renal failure should be introduced to renal specialists when the creatinine exceeds about 300 μmol/l.

**Dr AJC Pickering,
The Village Surgery**

Dear Charles

I would appreciate your advice about a man with diabetes and a slowly rising serum creatinine.

Rajesh Shah is a 60 year old retired teacher who developed diabetes six years ago. He takes glibenclamide 5 mg twice daily. His HbAlc is 9% and his blood pressure is controlled at 164/84 on an ACE inhibitor. He has no other complications of diabetes.

At Rajesh's last review, we checked his biochemistry and noted that his creatinine was 180 μmol/l compared with 140 six months ago and 115 this time last year. He has developed proteinuria, two plus on testing with Multistix, whereas all past tests have been negative for protein in the urine.

Rajesh has always shown an interest in the monitoring of his diabetes asking, for example, what we tested his urine for. He understands that diabetes can damage the kidneys and that such damage would be shown by a rising creatinine and proteinuria. His next door neighbour, a 56 year old with end-stage renal failure caused by chronic glomerulonephritis, is treated by peritoneal dialysis.

I would like to know, specifically, whether we should refer Rajesh to the renal unit, whether we should undertake further tests such as a creatinine clearance and an intravenous pyelogram, and the point at which continued treatment with ACE inhibitors might contribute to deteriorating renal function.

Yours sincerely

Tony

continue taking sulphonylureas. However, metformin should not be used in renal failure as it carries an increased risk of lactic acidosis, a potentially lethal complication.

Management of patients in chronic renal failure

These people need a lot of support. They have to cope with the prospect of dialysis/transplant and are at risk of other

**Dr Charles Fox, The Diabetes Centre,
District General Hospital**

Dear Tony
    Thank you for writing to me about Rajesh Shah. This is an unusual case and there are a number of features which mark Rajesh out from the typical patient who is entering the final phase of diabetic nephropathy.

    1.   No previous proteinuria
    There is normally a progression from microalbuminuria to Albustix-positive proteinuria with measurable renal failure developing several years later.
    2.   No other microvascular complications
    It is a rule that patients with established diabetic nephropathy invariably have some evidence of retinopathy. I have checked Rajesh's retinal photographs and they are free from any signs of retinal disease.
    3.   Rapid deterioration in renal function
    I have plotted the reciprocal of the three serum creatinine measurements against time and there is a linear deterioration in renal function. If this continues unabated, Rajesh's creatinine will exceed 500 μmol/l within the next 12 months.

    You do not mention when you started treatment with the ACE inhibitor, but if this took place within the last 18 months then this drug could be responsible for the deteriorating function. You should stop the ACE inhibitor and repeat the creatinine measurement in two weeks. An improvement in renal function would suggest the presence of a renal artery stenosis as a cause of Rajesh's hypertension. You should listen for renal bruits, looking for further evidence of this diagnosis. We should consider renal angiography to try and identify a narrowing of one or both renal arteries that could be correctable by angioplasty or surgery.
    If, on the other hand, Rajesh has been taking an ACE inhibitor for several years without any previous fall-off in renal function, the possibility of renal artery stenosis is small. To be on the safe side, it would still be worth withdrawing the ACE inhibitor for a month or so to see whether this leads to an improvement in serum creatinine. During this period, it would be sensible to use an alternative antihypertensive such as nifedipine.
    Assuming that withdrawal of the ACE inhibitor has no beneficial effect, it looks as if Rajesh has an aggressive renal disease which will require dialysis in the next year or so. As it is not a characteristic example of diabetic nephropathy, I would suggest early referral to the renal unit. I will be interested to hear whether they carry out a renal biopsy or any other investigations to make a positive diagnosis.
    Yours sincerely

complications which may still be undeclared. They should receive their care from a single person or, failing that, a team who can give a coherent account of the management plan. This person can of course be a GP who feels confident and competent to provide diabetes care.

In an ideal world as the renal failure progresses, the patient would attend a joint clinic with the nephrologist and diabetic specialist. This would facilitate the same smooth handover of care that routinely occurs in the transfer of young people with diabetes from the care of paediatricians to adult diabetologists. Unfortunately nephrologists are too thin on the ground to allow this luxury in the average district general hospital.

End stage renal failure (ESRF)

In the early 1980s it was unusual for patients with diabetes to receive renal replacement therapy, but thanks to the campaign waged by an enthusiastic nephrologist and the British Diabetic Association, patients with ESRF due to diabetes have the same chance of treatment as any patient dying of kidney disease.

By the time diabetes has caused ESRF, it has usually damaged other organs. Thus 72% of such patients had significant cardiac disease and in half of those it was severe, with over 70% coronary occlusion. A study organised by the British Diabetic Association found that 35% of patients with renal failure also had severe bilateral visual loss.

Haemodialysis

It is the rule that patients with ESRF have invariably suffered other ravages of diabetes and in particular have atheromatous peripheral vessels which hinders the formation of arteriovenous shunts to provide access for dialysis. This form of treatment is not usually the best option.

Chronic ambulatory peritoneal dialysis (CAPD)

When this was first introduced in the late 1970s, it was taken up with enthusiasm by patients who felt a release from being tied to a machine three times a week. Provided they could fit the dialysis bags into their car, they could travel freely. There is an ever-present risk of peritoneal infection and patients have to take meticulous care when changing bags.

CAPD has become routine in diabetes care, and there is the added advantage that insulin can be given into the peritoneal bag allowing absorption into the liver via the portal vein. This is a more physiological arrangement than injecting subcutaneously, when insulin reaches the liver after passage through the lungs. Like many good schemes, peritoneal insulin does not work in every case, but is worth a try.

Transplantation

Results from pioneering centres using live related donors have been encouraging, with 65% survival at five years. European figures transplanting cadaver donor kidneys have not been so impressive, with a survival rate of 49% at three years. Clearly the best quality of life for patients with ESRF must be a successful transplant with cyclosporin for immunosuppression.

Blood pressure is a normally distributed variable, affected by many pathological features, and influenced by the sight of white coats, exercise and anxiety. It is an everyday experience to be faced with decisions about blood pressure in our diabetic patients:

- On routine testing the patient has a markedly raised pressure. Should we check it a few days before starting treatment?
- Should we ask the patient who responds well to an ACE inhibitor to persevere despite the complaint of cough?
- How forcibly should we encourage drug therapy in the borderline hypertensive patient who is reluctant to comply?

It is interesting to try and predict how patients will react to the measurement of blood pressure. Many are so hardened that they barely notice the procedure and affect no interest in the result. Most people with raised pressure have well-tried defence mechanisms for explaining away a high value. "Stress" is a favourite and some play off the hospital against the GP or the practice nurse. This is an educational problem which we need to address.

Large population studies (e.g. from Bedford or Framingham) have shown an increased prevalence of hypertension in NIDDs

COMMANDMENT

Educate patients about the importance of BP in diabetes

TEACHING POINT

Patients should be told the meaning of systolic and diastolic pressure and the threshold for starting treatment in their particular case

compared with the normal population. Hypertension is even more common in IDDs, particularly if there is frank albuminuria or microalbuminuria, which highlights the link between hypertension and diabetic renal disease.

"Mild" hypertension is usually defined as a diastolic pressure of between 90 and 110. Several large studies have investigated the benefits of treating mild hyptertension in the non-diabetic population. Most trials have shown that treatment reduces the risk of stroke but not of cardiac events, with no reduction in the overall mortality. Thus, since the risk in diabetes seems much greater, parallel studies in patients with diabetes are needed.

The UK Prospective Diabetes Study (see Chapter 3) is examining the long term effects of different treatment regimens in 4400 patients with NIDDM. In the course of this study, it was found that 40% of men and over 50% of women also had hypertension. In view of this remarkably strong association, a randomised hypertension study was grafted onto the UKPDS. After four and a half years' follow-up, it appeared that the combined risks of hypertension and NIDDM were much greater

COMMANDMENT

Check BP annually in all patients – especially if there is proteinuria

than diabetes on its own (see Figure 14.1). For instance, the overall risk of a diabetes related death was 2.3% in the normotensive group and 5.3% in the group with hypertension. Hypertension was associated with a threefold increase in risk of amputation amd non-fatal stroke. The full study results will not be known until 1998, but in the meantime we can try to persuade our patients to give up smoking – a well recognised way of reducing the danger of a stroke.

In patients with established diabetic renal disease, effective blood pressure treatment can markedly reduce the rate of decline of renal function and reduce by half the urinary albumin loss.

Figure 14.1

Mortality and morbidity in normotensive and hypertensive patients over a median of 4.6 years' follow-up

EVENTS	Normotensive patients		Hypertensive patients	
	n 2203	%	n 1445	%
Cardiac deaths	40	1.8	52	3.6
Deaths from stroke	4	0.2	13	0.9
Non-fatal myocardial infarct	48	2.2	47	3.3
Non-fatal stroke	12	0.5	23	1.6
Amputation	4	0.2	8	0.6
Blindness	18	0.8	15	1.0

Dr AJC Pickering,
The Village Surgery

Dear Charles

I have a problem with poor control of hypertension in some of my patients with diabetes.

We know that in the general population, blood pressure in excess of 160/90 is one of the risk factors for ischaemic heart disease and stroke. The value to the individual of treating blood pressure rises with age and is more certain in respect of stroke than ischaemic heart disease. People with diabetes are at risk of cardiovascular disease in general and myocardial infarction in particular. Their risk of a stroke is up to three times that of the general population. We have shared this information with our patients and work with them towards some sort of control.

The problem for me is that I am not sure how tightly to control blood pressure for I am conscious that extra therapies are "add-on" problems for people with diabetes. I know of no firm evidence showing that control of hypertension protects against death from myocardial infarction in diabetes, though I believe the UKPDS is looking at this.

How would you answer my 72 year old patient, Peter Jefferson, who enjoys life, is free from ophthalmic and peripheral vascular complications, but who dreads my tinkering with his uncontrolled hypertension (182/104) because all the therapies I have tried make him feel terrible? He asked me today whether I was saving him from a heart attack in order to wait for and treat another potential problem? Certainly, should he develop peripheral vascular disease and become housebound, I would feel I had not served him well.

To complicate matters, the Health Authority are now fussing about the number of untreated or uncontrolled hypertensives registered with the practice. They seem to expect us to ensure that Peter Jefferson is treated.

Any thoughts?

Yours sincerely

Tony

**Dr Charles Fox, The Diabetes Centre,
District General Hospital**

Dear Tony

Thank you for your letter about Peter Jefferson, who sounds like the sort of patient who is really trying to understand the issues. He is clearly taking up a lot of your time but I am sure it will be rewarding. I will try to avoid jargon in my reply and you may want to copy my reply to Peter — provided you agree with the sentiments!

I will try to answer the following points:

1.   The relative increased risk in diabetes of strokes and heart disease.
2.   The benefits of treating high blood pressure in diabetes — both proven and assumed.
3.   Given the side-effects, is treatment of high blood pressure worth the candle?
4.   How can you square the decision of you and your patient with the Health Authority's ambition for the population as a whole?

The general figure bandied about is that people with diabetes have about twice the risk of developing heart disease and stroke. When you look at the original studies, the picture is much more confusing, with different risks affecting different populations. Thus if you are an inhabitant of Framingham (a small town in America) diabetes causes a threefold risk of having a stroke, while in Japan there seems to be no increased risk of stroke attached to diabetes. You mention the UKPDS: preliminary results of this study suggest that if you develop diabetes later in life, raised blood pressure doubles the risk of serious disease of the arteries, i.e. heart attacks, strokes or amputation. From most of the evidence it appears that, in diabetes, the risks of stroke vs heart disease are about equal and there is some evidence emerging that in diabetes high blood pressure increases the risk of developing retinopathy, which of course is one of the great concerns of people living with diabetes.

In the 1970s and 80s a number of long-term studies were set up to answer the question "Do patients with raised blood pressure benefit from treatment?" A great deal of time, money and organisation went into these trials, the largest of which included 17,000 patients who were studied for over five years. Each trial came up with slightly different answers. Overall, however, they showed that treating slightly raised blood pressure halved the risk of stroke but had very little effect on heart disease. We can only guess whether the same results will apply to a diabetic population. There are some reasons for thinking that the the benefits may be greater in diabetes and we hope that the UKPDS will come up with a clear answer.

However, there is the added factor of kidney disease. You don't mention whether Peter Jefferson has any protein in his urine to suggest that his kidneys are affected by diabetes. If so, there is plenty of evidence that controlling his blood pressure will slow down the damage to his kidneys. In fact some specialists are recommending that patients with early kidney damage take an ACE inhibitor even if their blood pressure is normal because this group of drugs, which effectively control blood pressure, also protect the kidneys from diabetic injury.

The treatment of high blood pressure would be a simple matter if it weren't for the side-effects of the drugs we use. Most patients visit their doctor with some complaint – usually pain or disability. The sort of blood pressure you have measured in Peter causes no symptoms and he will feel perfectly well until he takes the tablets you prescribe. It is up to your pharmacological skills to find the best therapy for Peter and, in his turn, he must be patient and give your medication the benefit of the doubt. In difficult cases, there must be commitment on both sides to arrive at optimum therapy. If Peter is keen to reduce his blood pressure, there are non-pharmacological manoeuvres which may help. If he smokes, he can greatly reduce his risk of arterial disease by giving up.

I am sorry you are feeling threatened by the Health Authority – I always thought you had them eating out of your hand. There seem to be two sorts of edicts from on high that doctors are learning to live with: (a) demands that we see twice as many patients without keeping them waiting and with half the resources, and (b) clinical demands with which you disagree on professional grounds. Fortunately we can still put our side of the argument and I can't see the Health Authority penalising you if the patient is fully informed and decides not to take the treatment offered.

I look forward to hearing what decision you and Peter come to about his blood pressure.

Yours sincerely

BLOOD PRESSURE MEASUREMENT

How to measure BP

- Take it seriously – you may start lifelong treatment on the strength of two BP readings
- Calibrate electronic machines every six months

COMMANDMENT

Treat raised blood pressure more aggressively in patients with early evidence of renal disease

- Check the tubing and connection
- Use the right sized cuff – a large cuff is necessary if the circumference of the arm exceeds 33 cm
- Take the diastolic at phase 5 (5th sound – when the sound vanishes completely)

Threshold for treatment

The threshold for treatment is 160/95 for patients in their fifties and 160/100 for those in their sixties. Patients aged under 50 may warrant treatment if their BP is above 140/90, particularly if there is any measurable degree of renal involvement.

MANAGEMENT

Every article on hypertension stresses the importance of non-pharmacological measures before wading in with drugs. Patients with diabetes are already making changes to their lifestyle in response to one disease and they may be reluctant to make any further concessions. If they have ignored advice to stop smoking because of diabetes, they are unlikely to summon up the necessary willpower on account of hypertension. The same applies to alcohol and weight reduction. Perhaps the doctor and patient can salve their consciences by avoiding added salt in their diet.

Patients with raised blood pressure should have their electrolytes measured. They also need an ECG and chest X-ray to assess the degree of left ventricular hypertrophy.

Secondary causes of hypertension are rare in practice, but one should think of:

- Cushing's syndrome (characteristic appearance)
- Phaeochromocytoma (variable BP, headaches, sweating, rage)
- Hyperaldosteronism (hypokalaemia)

Target blood pressure

Aim at a stable BP of 140/90 and tell the patient this at the outset of treatment.

COMMANDMENT

Measure the diastolic pressure at the point when the audible impulse ends (5th sound)

COMMANDMENT

Aim for a target BP of 140/90, with concessions to age

The following factors may affect your decisions about the treatment of blood pressure:

- The attitude of the patient
- The presence of retinopathy
- Nephropathy, either microalbuminuria or Albustix-positive albuminuria

COMMANDMENT
Check the fundi if BP is raised

Resistance to treatment

This may present a dilemma, especially amongst young people who are often reluctant to address the problem. Coping with diabetes takes up all the time/energy they can devote to medical concerns. Their attitude to maintaining their blood pressure at an appropriate level may be: "Not another thing for me to worry about".

Pharmaceutical treatment

Patients whose blood pressure levels persist over the age-related threshold for treatment will need to be prescribed antihypertensive agents. There are five main groups of drugs are used in the management of raised BP – thiazides, loop diuretics, beta blockers, calcium antagonists and ACE inhibitors. Alpha blockers and methyldopa may also have a role

COMMANDMENT
Recheck mildly raised BP over three months before starting treatment

COMMANDMENT
Remember all antihypertensive agents have side-effects

Figure 14.2

Antihypertensive agents

	Advantages	Drawbacks
Thiazides e.g. bendrofluazide 2.5 mg daily	Inexpensive	Orthostatic hypotension Slow-acting in the elderly Diabetogenic Hypokalaemia (trivial with indapamide) May precipitate hyperosmolar coma Impotence May precipitate gout Need to monitor serum potassium
Loop diuretics e.g. frusemide 20 mg daily	Inexpensive	Drastic diuresis – often inconvenient Hypokalaemia
Beta blockers e.g. atenolol 100 mg daily	Slow action In angina, protects from sudden death (mild effect)	Vasoconstriction Excerbation of asthma Lipid status worsened Blunt warning of hypos
Ca antagonists e.g. nifedipine LA 30 mg daily	Peripheral vasodilation May help in angina Ankle oedema	Headaches Flushing
ACE inhibitors e.g. captopril 25 mg bd	May lessen proteinuria Best in "quality of life" studies	Renal failure in presence of unilateral renal disease – renal failure is quite common in old people with diabetes First dose hypotension Expensive
Others Alpha blockers e.g. doxazocine 1 mg daily	Improve impotence	
Methyldopa	When all else fails	

in some cases. However, the decision over when to start such treatment and which line of treatment to pursue must be taken with care as all such drugs have potential side-effects (see Figure 14.2).

Best buy

ACE inhibitors are certainly not the cheapest antihypertensive agents, but there is good reason to make them first line treatment in diabetes. They deliver benefit in renal disease in addition to lowering blood pressure, and come out well in quality of life studies. In practice, ACE inhibitors are a safe group of drugs but should be used with knowledge of the problems:

COMMANDMENT
Monitor renal function regularly in patients taking ACE inhibitors

1. **Cough**.
   This troubles up to 10% of patients, and those patients will be intolerant of all ACE inhibitors. It can sometimes be suppressed by adding the non-steroidal sulindac 200 mg bd.

2. **Renal failure**
   This may be induced by ACE inhibitors in patients with renal artery stenosis, who rely on renin to maintain perfusion of the kidney. Baseline renal function should be measured before starting an ACE inhibitor and again two weeks later.

3.   **Severe hypotension**

Patients who have been taking high doses of diuretics have raised levels of angiotensin, and ACE inhibitors should be used with caution as they may cause a dramatic fall in blood pressure.

4.   **Hyperkalaemia**

A potential risk, which means that loop diuretics complement ACE inhibitors. The latter should not be used in combination with potassium-sparing diuretics.

CORONARY HEART DISEASE

HOW COMMON IS HEART DISEASE IN DIABETES?

Most of the population studies discussed below lump together IDDM and NIDDM and therefore relate mainly to NIDDM, the more common form of diabetes.

The Framingham study (1979) came out with the bald statement that the incidence of cardiovascular disease among diabetic men was twice that of non-diabetic men and among diabetic women, the risk was three times that of non-diabetic women. The reason for the gender difference is that non-diabetic women before the menopause are protected from cardiovascular disease and diabetic women lose this protection.

Having established that diabetes is a risk factor for coronary heart disease (CHD), it would help to know whether the excess risk is due simply to the raised blood glucose or whether the other risk factors which cluster with diabetes (hypertension, obesity, hypercholesterolaemia, microalbuminuria) are the main culprits. Since the various studies are planned using different criteria and populations, it is not surprising that the detailed results tend to be confusing. However, a few key points emerge:

1.   Heart disease is the main cause of death in diabetes

In 1979, a study was set up to examine the death certificates of people with diabetes who died under the age of 50. Four hundred and forty-eight cases were identified, and the single most common cause of death was CHD, which accounted for 31% of the total. In an older population, this percentage would be even higher.

2.   The excess risk applies even to those with marginally elevated blood glucose levels

In a 15 year mortality study of Whitehall civil servants, the relative risk of dying from CHD was 1.4 in those with impaired glucose tolerance and 2.7 in those with full-blown diabetes.

3.   The cardiac risk factors are cumulative

This principle has been established in the non-diabetic population. Thus smoking, hypercholesterolaemia and hypertension appear to be independent risk factors, each one adding to the risk of a person developing CHD. The same risk factors apply in diabetes but the graph is shifted upwards so that the overall risk is approximately double.

4.   So far no prospective study shows that tight diabetic control reduces the risk of CHD

The DCCT (see Chapter 3) was designed to investigate small vessel disease in a group of young adults from North America. Few cases of myocardial infarction were seen throughout the study. The UKPDS is investigating the effect of different treatment regimens on the development of small and large vessel disease. The main cohort of patients with NIDDM have been recruited since 1982 and no firm conclusions are expected until 1998.

5. Patients with or without diabetes should stop smoking

By using meta-analysis, it has been shown that stopping smoking is better than any other intervention and would prolong by three years the life of the average 45 year old man with diabetes.

ASPIRIN

This simple substance has been shown to have remarkable properties in reducing the risk of recurrence in acute myocardial infarction, transient ischaemic attack from carotid artery atheroma and cerebral thrombosis. The relevant trials have been carried out in the non-diabetic population, but there is no reason to suppose that the effect of aspirin on platelet stickiness is not equally effective in diabetes. People with diabetes are also at risk of the complications of aspirin prophylaxis, namely gastric ulceration. Only 75 mg ("a quarter of an aspirin") daily is needed.

SYNDROME X

Syndrome X is the name used by diabetologists to describe a constellation of symptoms which commonly coincide. (NB cardiologists use "Syndrome X" to describe the condition in which a patient has classical symptoms of angina and whistle-clean coronary arteries as demonstrated on angiogram.) Our

Syndrome X was described by Reavan and consists of:

- Insulin resistance
- Hyperinsulinaemia
- Glucose intolerance
- Hypertension
- Central obesity
- Increased VLDL triglyceride
- Decreased HDL cholesterol

Many NIDDs present this pattern of abnormalities and the combination of hypertension and lipid imbalance conspires to lay down atheroma. These patients are at serious risk of cardio-vascular disease and the key to solving the problem is weight loss. Unfortunately, this may be impossible to maintain. We are faced with a number of conflicting options:

- Improving diabetic control with sulphonylureas or insulin leads to increased body weight
- Controlling blood pressure with thiazide diuretics increases the blood glucose
- Beta blockers for hypertension decrease HDL cholesterol

CLINICAL MANAGEMENT OF CARDIAC DISEASE IN DIABETES

Heart disease does not require any unconventional treat-ment in diabetes. Take seriously any complaint of pain in the chest, arm or jaw. Ask about the classic associations of exer-cise, cold weather and exertion on a full stomach. Now that coronary angiography has become routine, we know that many patients with CHD never experience the textbook symptoms and doctors must maintain a high index of suspicion. Some believe that all patients over 40 years of age should have an annual ECG. This is probably not a good idea since, in the UK, anti-anginal drugs are only prescribed in patients with symptoms. On the other hand, a therapeutic trial of a vasodilator (glyceryl trinitrate inhaler or buccal Suscard) will often help with the diagnosis.

If the history suggests angina and the ECG is normal, an exercise ECG will often provide evidence of ischaemic heart disease. If the story of angina is not typical and the exercise test is negative, significant coronary disease is unlikely.

Treatment of angina

Start with a long-acting nitrate with the usual warnings about headache. The next move would be the addition of a beta blocker. Patients on insulin need to be alerted to the possibility that their usual warning of hypos will be altered by these drugs. They should not be used in patients with asthma or peripheral vascular disease. Beta blockers may cause cold hands and feet and lead to erectile failure. They act by reducing the force and frequency of cardiac contraction and may precipitate dizziness or left ventricular failure.

Diabetes should not be a deterrent to coronary bypass surgery and this should be considered in any patient whose angina persists despite full medical treatment.

Myocardial infarction

Not only is heart disease much more common, but also the mortality of myocardial infarction is doubled in patients with diabetes. The main cause of this excess mortality is pump failure (cardiogenic shock or intractable congestive cardiac failure), presumably because the acute infarction has often occurred on a background of widespread "small vessel" disease of the coronary arteries. People with diabetes are also at greater risk of dying suddenly before they ever reach the coronary care unit. This sudden death may be due to arrhythmia, though there is no obvious reason why this should be more common in diabetes.

Dr AJC Pickering,
The Village Surgery

Dear Charles

We are trying to sort out a practice protocol for people with diabetes and I would value your opinion on the following points concerning screening for CHD risk factors.

Some of my colleagues ask diabetic patients to have an ECG annually. In our practice of 4500 patients, 86 of whom have diabetes, this would involve our practice nurse in about 50 hours of extra work a year. Given that there is a false negative in the use of ECGs to diagnose coronary heart disease, we do not feel that this is a good use of practice nurse time. What are your views on the subject?

We measure serum lipid levels of all people with diabetes at the time of diagnosis and then every five years or so. Regardless of their lipid profile, we advise all people with diabetes to moderate their intake of animal fats, take regular exercise and avoid smoking. Is this a reasonable compromise, taking into consideration the costs involved?

It would be helpful if we might accord some priority to the risk factors for CHD in people without symptoms of the problem. We propose the following (in descending order of priority):

1. Smoking
2. Lack of exercise
3. Hypertension
4. Obesity (BMI >30)
5. Hyperlipidaemia

The intention is that we should focus on smoking before worrying about serum lipids, but that we would not fail to offer treatment or advice about a low priority factor if there were no prospect of improving others of higher priority. Would you comment on our "hit list"?

Yours sincerely

Tony

**Dr Charles Fox, The Diabetes Centre,
District General Hospital**

Dear Tony

I like the careful structure you have set up for diabetes care in your practice. Good organisation is an essential component of a service which will satisfy our patients and achieve the aims set by the St Vincent Declaration. It should be easier to manage change effectively in a GP practice than in the unwieldy juggernaut of a hospital clinic.

I was not aware that GP colleagues arrange annual ECGs as a routing screening test, though this is certainly done in some hospital clinics. We carry out routine ECGs in the setting of the UKPDS research clinic where cardiovascular disease is an important end-point. Many patients have minor ECG changes and, in a few cases, the ECG shows definite ischaemic changes even though careful questioning fails to elicit any symptoms. As you point out, the converse may also apply, with undoubted angina in the presence of a normal ECG.

It is not current practice in the UK to treat cardiac ischaemia in the absence of symptoms and we can only watch these patients with concern and some trepidation. At the first sign of chest pain, we give anti-angina therapy and consider exercise testing.

Until such a day as it becomes standard practice to treat asymptomatic coronary heart disease, I would not recommend routing ECG screening outside the context of research. It is not included in the British Diabetic Association Patients' Charter "What Care to Expect". Of course, we must be open to the possibility of CHD in people coming to the Diabetic Clinic and investigate fully patients with angina or hypertension.

Lipid measurements are a difficult issue in diabetes care. At the time of diagnosis, triglyceride levels are often raised and it is best to postpone the first lipid profile until good (or the best possible) control of blood glucose has been achieved. If the results are normal, it is reasonable to check lipids after an arbitrary time lapse of five years.

I like your hit list of priorities for risk factors. The responsibility for at least three out of the five lies entirely with the patient. We hope that the UKPDS will help us decide how aggressively to treat hypertension in NIDDs, but there is good evidence for keeping blood pressure below 140/85 in those with any degree of renal involvement.

Yours sincerely

Another event which occurs more frequently in diabetes is a "silent infarct". It is well documented that a routine ECG may show convincing evidence of a previous myocardial infarction while the patient denies ever suffering the expected symptoms. This phenomenon of a "silent infarction" occurs more commonly in diabetes. From a practical point of view, any diabetic patient who is distressed, with a slow pulse rate, low blood pressure or an arrythmia, deserves an urgent ECG.

The stress of a heart attack invariably puts up the blood glucose and it might be hoped that keeping the blood glucose normal would reduce the excess risk. Unfortunately this has not been borne out by clinical trials but, in the high-tech environment of a coronary care unit, it is sensible to keep the blood glucose normal with an intravenous insulin pump.

A diabetic patient with a myocardial infarct should receive conventional treatment. In particular, streptokinase is used according to the normal criteria. Diabetic retinopathy is listed as a contraindication to thrombolysis, but this only applies in the presence of active new vessel formation. If retinopathy has been successfully treated, there should be no excess risk of haemorrhage.

COMMANDMENT

Remember that 75% of deaths in NIDDM are due to coronary heart disease

TEACHING POINT

Unlike small vessel disease, the duration of diabetes does not have major impact on the risk of coronary heart disease

Acute stroke

As with heart disease, cerebrovascular disease is at least twice as common in diabetes, and the fatality rate after an acute stroke is also doubled in patients with known diabetes.

The stress of a cerebrovascular accident may cause a significant rise in plasma glucose and it is important to know whether the patient had previously undiagnosed diabetes. If so, the HbA1c should also be raised, whereas it will be normal if the hyperglycaemia is a recent, and hopefully transient, reaction to the biological insult of a stroke.

There is some evidence that good control of blood glucose improves the outcome following a stroke, presumably because a raised blood glucose level increases the area of cerebral ischaemia.

Hyperlipidaemia

People with diabetes have so many restrictions on their lifestyle and diet that it seems hard to introduce another problem into their lives.

The British Diabetic Association's Patients' Charter "What Care to Expect" recommends that "blood fats are checked at least once per year". This would present to the biochemistry labs of the UK an additional three quarter of a million samples per annum and would increase the sum of human unhappiness without saving many lives. (Professor John Yudkin of Univer-sity College Hospital calculated that it would be necessary to treat a notional middle-aged diabetic man with hypercholesterolaemia for 803 years to prevent a single death from CHD.)

In diabetic as in non-diabetic subjects the risk of cardiovascular disease is directly proportional to LDL cholesterol and inversely proportional to HDL cholesterol. Hypertriglyceridaemia is commonly found in NIDDM but is probably not an independent risk factor for heart disease.

**Dr AJC Pickering,
The Village Surgery**

Dear Charles

I would value your advice about Winston Guidon, a 52 year old from Trinidad, who has had NIDDM for two years. The dilemma is how far to investigate his cardiovascular system.

Winston's diabetes is well-controlled on glibenclamide 5 mg twice daily, as assessed by an HbA1c of 7.5% and the absence of complications in the eyes, the feet and the kidneys. However, he does have hypertension (BP 170/94, taking enalapril 20 mg daily and frusemide 20 mg daily), and has symptoms compatible with angina or reflux oesophagitis. He is overweight (BMI 32) with a large belly. He no longer smokes but, until the diagnosis of diabetes and since his teens, he had smoked about ten cigarettes daily.

He suffers a moderately severe pain – centrally in the chest radiating to the neck – from time to time. This is unrelated to exercise or posture in any consistent way. He has a burning discomfort in the chest if he drinks hot liquids. He belches a lot and is short of breath walking uphill. On examination, he has a bit of epigastric tenderness. A recent ECG reported as normal. We referred him for gastroscopy and he has moderate oesophagitis. We worked our way through appropriate remedies for this problem, from antacids through cimetidine and ranitidine to omeprazole, but the symptoms, though improved slightly, remain. He has a strong family history of heart disease, his father and two brothers having had heart attacks in their late fifties.

I think he has oesophagitis and atypical angina. Certainly he is at risk of premature death.

How far should I pursue investigations? Would a normal exercise ECG test be that reassuring? How, were the exercise test to be normal, do we justify to him the risks of angiography? He is somewhat anxious, in general, and I would not wish to give him the message, by rigorous investigation, that he is doomed to the same fate as his brothers.

I am tempted to suggest an exercise ECG and then call a halt but take out an insurance in the form of aspirin prophylaxis. What do you think?

Yours aye

Tony

**Dr Charles Fox, The Diabetes Centre,
District General Hospital**

Dear Tony

Thank you for asking me about Winston.

Atypical chest pain is a common problem and a number of such patients are admitted as emergencies. If the pain is severe enough to warrant a hospital stay, we usually keep the patients in for a few days to check serial ECGs and cardiac enzymes. Provided that these tests rule out the possibility of a myocardial infarction, we discharge the patients home and treat them in a similar way to your management of Winston. We too have patients with oesophagitis, demonstrated at gastroscopy, whose symptoms fail to improve on omeprazole. Given the effectiveness of H2 antagonists, this strongly suggests that the pain does not originate from the oesophagus.

In the pre-coronary angiogram era, cardiology textbooks included a whole chapter on angina describing in great detail the subtle nuances in the history which could only be obtained by a skilled cardiologist. Now coronary angiography has become routine, it is apparent that true cardiac pain is often atypical.

Winston certainly needs an exercise test. If he completes the full 12 minutes of the Bruce protocol and achieves his predicted maximal heart rate without chest pain, he could be reassured that his cardiac function was up to the mark. People who perform as well as this in an exercise test have a low risk of developing significant cardiac events, whether or not they have coronary heart disease. Thus a normal exercise test would reduce the need for coronary angiography.

In practice Winston, with his impressive BMI, is not likely to achieve a high exercise workload. Coronary angiography is easily available, and most cardiologists would be happy to proceed, particularly if the exercise test revealed ischaemic ST changes.

I can understand why Winston is anxious about all this attention on his heart. However, coronary disease is really a mechanical problem with the patient paying a high price if we make the wrong decisions. Chest pain itself is a worrying symptom but he would be reassured if his exercise test or coronary angiogram were normal. On the other hand he might turn out to be a candidate for coronary bypass surgery. Either way, he might escape the fate of his father and brothers.

Yours sincerely

WHEN THINKING ABOUT LIPIDS ASK ABOUT OTHER RISK FACTORS:

- What is the patient's smoking history, now or in the past?

- Any past history of heart disease?

- Any chest pain suggestive of angina?

- Any family history of heart disease or stroke?

- Is the blood pressure raised?

- Is there proteinuria or microalbuminuria?

What lipid abnormalities occur in diabetes?

Abbreviations

VLDL	very low density lipoprotein
LDL	low density lipoprotein
HDL	high density lipoprotein
triG	triglyceride

Serum lipids in IDDM are likely to be abnormal only when the IDDM is untreated or poorly controlled:

- Marked triG, raised LDL-chol, low HDL-chol

Insulin corrects all these abnormalities.

NIDDM is associated with a raised triG, a raised VLDL, a normal LDL and a reduced HDL. Diet, together with sulphonylureas or insulin, corrects the first two abnormalities but has little effect on HDL cholesterol.

High VLDL and low HDL cholesterol are associated with central obesity, and a waist/hip ratio >1.

In addition, two rare specific lipid abnormalities may be associated with diabetes. Both of these conditions lead to xanthoma, a yellowish skin which is found in characteristic sites:

1. **Type V** (xanthoma scattered all over trunk, a bit like chicken pox) which results in very high triG levels of up to 30 mmol/l

   This is more than ten times the normal of less than 2.0. This does not seem to lead to increased heart disease, but may cause recurrent bouts of pancreatitis. If so, it may respond to large doses of fish oils (Maxepa).

2. **Type III** (xanthoma on knees and elbows with yellow striae on the palms of the hands) which presents with a raised cholesterol and triG

   There is a characteristic appearance on lipoprotein electrophoresis. These patients also run the risk of acute pancreatitis and often need a fibrate in addition to good control of their diabetes.

Screening for lipid abnormalities

Many centres follow the British Diabetic Association guidelines and screen serum lipids every year as part of the annual review. This is a simple solution and the easiest to organise. Because triglycerides are important in diabetes, it is necessary to obtain blood after a 14 hour fast and measure total cholesterol and triglyceride as well as LDL and HDL cholesterol.

In patients with IDDM, lipids should be measured once good metabolic control has been achieved. If the results are completely normal, there is no point in repeating them until five years later. If they are borderline, however, the process should be repeated at the next annual review. Abnormal results should be treated with dietary advice in the first instance.

The policy in NIDDM should be to aim at identifying those patients with hyperlipidaemia who are likely to benefit from treatment; for instance, patients under the age of 65 who have any history of heart disease or who admit to symptoms of angina and a family history of CHD. Patients with hypertension and/or proteinuria should be screened. It is a moot point whether to screen those patients who increase their risk of CHD by smoking.

Should lipid disorders be treated differently in diabetes?

Several studies have shown that lowering plasma lipid levels reduces the risk of CHD in non-diabetic subjects and is particulary effective after coronary bypass grafting. It is worth noting, however, that the total morbidity was unchanged in the group receiving active treatment. There have been no trials of lipid lowering agents in diabetes. In the absence of definite proof though, it seems reasonable to treat patients in the normal way.

Aims of treatment

The aims of treatment are as follows:

■   To keep LDL cholesterol <3.5 mmol/l
■   To keep HDL cholesterol >1.0 mmol/l

Treatment strategy

There is a tendency for doctors, both in hospital and in general practice, when faced with abnormal lipids to start wondering which would be the best drug to correct the problem. However, it is vital to regard nutritional changes as the key. This may not go down well with patients as nobody likes to change their eating habits and it is more attractive to imagine that a little pill would be the best way of putting things right. However, lipid lowering agents are not particularly potent; the most effective will only reduce LDL levels by 30% and increase HDL by 20%.

Patient education

This should be tailored to the individual. However, the main messages are likely to include some or all of the following:

- Stop smoking
- Take exercise, which reduces triglycerides and increases HDL-cholesterol
- Combat excess weight by restricting calories
- Limit dietary cholesterol
- Restrict saturated fatty acids
- Restrict total fat to <30% total calories
- Aim at taking 50–60% of calories from carbohydrate

Lipid lowering agents

These should be considered if, after a period of dieting, LDL cholesterol is >4.1 mmol/l. A fasting triglyceride level above 4–6 mmol/l carries a risk of pancreatitis and warrants drug therapy.

Lipid lowering agents are listed in Figure 15.1. All can be used in diabetes, although there is a theoretical difficulty with bile acid sequestrants which may exacerbate hypertriglyceridaemia.

Since many lipid lowering agents cause gastrointestinal side-effects, their use may be limited in patients already taking metformin or acarbose. Once drug therapy has been initiated, combinations of drugs may be needed to achieve the desired target.

If cholesterol and triglycerides are both raised, first line therapy is a fibric acid derivative. If LDL cholesterol alone is raised, try either a fibrate or an HMG CoA reductase inhibitor.

Figure 15.1

List of lipid lowering agents

- Bile acid sequestrants, e.g. cholestyramine
- Fibric acid derivates, e.g. bezafibrate, fenofibrate, gemfibrozil
- HMG CoA reductase inhibitors, e.g. pravastatin, simvastatin
- Nicotinic acid derivates, e.g. acipimox

HORMONE REPLACEMENT THERAPY

Following the menopause, non-diabetic women are at risk of two major medical problems:

1. Cardiovascular disease

Women lose their pre-menopausal protection from heart attack, and their incidence of coronary disease is the same as in men of the same age.

2. Osteoporosis

This is defined as loss of bone mass. It commonly occurs in women around the time of the menopause.

In addition, many women experience the classical symptoms of the climacteric, such as hot flushes, headache and muscle pains.

Oestrogen replacement reduces the risk of CHD in post-menopausal women, possibly by improving the lipid profile (lower LDL, higher HDL cholesterol). It also slows down the rate of bone loss and has been shown to reduce the risk of subsequent fracture. In women with an intact uterus, oestrogen on its own carries a significant risk of endometrial cancer and needs to be combined with a progestogen.

In diabetes, there is no specific evidence that oestrogen reduces the already high risk of CHD. In the absence of definite proof, it is reasonable to give patients the benefit of the doubt and recommend HRT – at least this will help the hot flushes. There is also doubt as to whether osteoporosis is more common in women with diabetes. However, women at risk should certainly be offered HRT.

A large selection of different HRT preparations is available in different forms – cutaneous patches, tablets and implants. All are effective and each has its own pros and cons. It is best to discuss the options with the patient and let her make the choice.

Certain people with IDDM have a high risk of developing other "autoimmune" disease because of their genetic make-up. Unfortunately genetic profiles can only be measured in the context of research so we have to rely on screening those at predictable risk, while maintaining a high index of suspicion.

Vitiligo is the name for well-circumscribed depigmented areas of skin, usually on the face or hands. This is commonly found in people with autoimmune endocrine disorders such as IDDM and thyroid disease.

Thyroid disease is the most common autoimmune disorder to be linked with diabetes. Nearly 20% of young IDDs have thyroid autoantibodies, and 7% of these are hypothyroid and 1% thyrotoxic. Thus the prevalence of thyroid disease in this age group is between 1 and 2%.

It is hard to know whether to advise regular screening for thyroid disease in this group. Paediatricians usually carry out annual thyroid checks since undiagnosed hypothyroidism may result in a child who is permanently undersized. In older children, it might be logical to arrange a one-off screen for thyroid autoantibodies and proceed to regular biochemical tests in those who are positive. However, thyroid disease can occur without autoantibodies being present. Gastric parietal cell antibodies could be measured at the same time to identify patients at risk of pernicious anaemia.

The telltale sign of hypothyroidism is unexplained weight increase and this should be a trigger to check thyroid function. If you see the person in question frequently, don't be dismayed if you fail to spot the signs of hypothyroidism. The diagnosis is most commonly made by someone who has not been in contact with the patient for a year or so, and who may be struck by the change in appearance.

Rarely Addison's disease will coincide with diabetes. This is difficult to diagnose and not easy to treat. You should think of it in patients who are losing weight, pigmented and having frequent hypos. Blood pressure will be low and serum electrolytes abnormal, with low sodium and raised potassium levels.

THE DOCTOR AS TEACHER

17

The traditional attitude of the doctor as an "adult", paternal figure, compared with the patient as "child" in the doctor-patient relationship, may result in conflict, mistrust and dissatisfaction whenever the patient suffers chronic disease. Neither party feels comfortable and, more important, where progress exists at all it is both painful and slow.

The desirable end result, from either perspective, is an improvement in health. The patient's interest in this is implicit, and it is the *raison d'être* of the doctor.

It has been said that patients care about five outcomes of illness: pain, anxiety, disfigurement, disability and death. Patients with diabetes are threatened by all five of these, and the challenge to their ability to cope may be severe. Thus, although the doctor and patient have a shared goal in maintaining and improving health, the patient whose doctor dictates and scolds can hardly be blamed for poor compliance, rebellion or denial.

In any consultation there are two experts, the doctor expert in the disease and the patient expert in the experience of illness. Mutual respect, from which follows an exchange between adults, is fundamental to good communication. Each party is eager and able, unfettered by irritation, to learn from the other. Each is able to accept, without necessarily agreeing with, the other's view.

As doctors or nurses we have information and skills which we owe, as a matter of duty, to our patients. We could, by starting from an attitude of respect which allows a refusal to accept our opinion, use those skills and that knowledge where it is wanted. In so doing, the quality of education improves. With this improvement comes compliance, since one of the objectives of learning is to change behaviour. Conversely, if there is no compliance, then either the information is understood but rejected (the right of any adult in a discussion), or the educational process is deficient. In this case we as teachers should review the delivery of information. Thus there may be either a stalemate, accepted by both sides, or the challenge to alter the method of education

Eventually, most patients settle for whatever level of understanding and mastery they can manage, and often this will be less than the doctor hoped for. Coaxing patients towards greater understanding, more self-reliance, is difficult and frustrating. This is the doctor's challenge – and when we feel tempted to complain about its difficulty it does not always help to recall the greater challenge faced by the patient.

Another general difficulty in the care of chronic illness is that whenever patients stall in their progress, we may need to make an extra effort to clear the hurdle. Worse, we may have to break ingrained habits and ask open questions which invite patients to set the agenda for the consultation, and to take their time about it. Since GPs ration the care they deliver principally by rationing the time available to each patient, this is a formidable challenge indeed. Whereas the investment of time probably pays handsome dividends in the long term, it is often difficult in the short term not to resent the patient who needs more time than others in the same predicament.

Perhaps we should view the non-compliant, stubborn patient who "will not do as we say" not only as a challenge in a complex game but as an example of the richness of human variation, a friend with whom we agree to disagree. Then life can be fun after all, even in the diabetic clinic.

DILEMMAS FOR PATIENTS AND CARERS

18

In *Diabetes At Your Fingertips*, Sönksen, Fox and Judd used questions frequently asked by people with diabetes to cover areas of particular importance. Here, we have selected a number of those questions, reproduced the original answers and offer some further comment to highlight dilemmas perceived by patients or their carers.

We feel strongly that there are absolutes in diabetes care, hence the distinction between our "Commandments" and the text of this book. Pointedly, there are no commandments in this chapter, only opinions.

> **The majority of the questions here relate to IDDM. The selection is deliberate even though the majority of patients with diabetes are NIDDs. The aim of this section is to consider areas of concern not covered elsewhere in this book, including some that are uncommon.**

Since I was diagnosed I have been very depressed. Is there any link between depression and diabetes?

People vary very greatly in their mental response to developing diabetes. Some lucky ones take to their new condition easily, while others, like yourself, find the whole thing very depressing.

The depression seems to take two forms. At first, shock and even anger at the very outset coupled with fear of injections and the unspoken fear of complications. A few weeks later comes the depressing realisation that diabetes is for life, and not just a temporary disease which can be "cured". This type of depression seems to affect young people who are worried and are feeling insecure about the future.

A few people with diabetes feel that, in some way, they are imperfect, especially if they have previously been fitness fanatics. The best way round this feeling of inadequacy is to throw yourself into sporting activities with great enthusiasm. Exercise is good for all of us and people with diabetes have managed to reach the top in most forms of sport from ocean racing to international football.

If you treat your diabetes in a positive way rather than letting the condition control you, the depression will gradually lift.

The question concerns possible differences in the meaning of "depression" and whether this feeling is directly due to the chronic disease or is an indirect psychological consequence. In medicine, the term depression is distinguished from feelings such as resentment or sadness by the association with other specific symptoms. This is not the case in lay usage. Clinical depression can be treated by psychological methods or drugs. Where lay "depression" is, for example, anger, the better approach is through education and psychology. The confusion of causality with coincidence is also a problem, certainly for our patients but also for us as professionals. The "dilemma" lies in the assessment of the "depression", and therefore the management options, and in the uncertainty both of the assessment and of causality.

The problem would seem to be that the patient's response to the diagnosis is at variance with our view of how we ourselves might behave in similar circumstances, a view coloured by our freedom from the condition and our desire to minimise the potential complications. We would like the patient to be compliant to the model of behaviour we have come to believe is correct. We can understand his attitude, because we know it exists, but can we really feel with and for him? Should we even put ourselves in the role of the provider of solutions or would we do better to take the view that the problem being his, the solution should be his too?

One option is to introduce the patient to a group of similar people and trust that the mysterious forces working in group dynamics will allow him to modify his attitude by picking up ideas from other members in the group, including health advisers, tailoring his solution to his own mind set. This approach has been successful in other areas such as weight loss and smoking cessation, at least for some members of the group.

Is there any way of knowing how much extra Actrapid Insulin to give depending on my blood glucose level so I can maintain a better blood glucose?

The answer is yes, but it will require some experimenting on your part. The particular dose and type of insulin most suited to you can best be judged by repeated measurements of your body's response to the insulin you are taking. If you find, for example, that your blood glucose always goes high after breakfast then you may be able to prevent this by taking more Actrapid before breakfast, but before making any adjustments in insulin dosage it is important to see that the blood glucose changes you see are part of a regular pattern. This is part of the process of balancing insulin, diet and exercise, and we would caution against taking an extra dose of insulin if you come across a rather high blood glucose reading as an isolated finding. It is usually far better to try to work out a routine whereby you can prevent your blood glucose from rising too high rather than to take an extra injection of insulin after it has happened. There are exceptions to this rule, of course. If you suddenly become unwell and your blood glucose goes very high, repeated extra injections of a short-acting insulin such as Actrapid are the most effective way of preventing the development of ketoacidosis.

Here the problem is that good control demands both experience and careful observation, hard work rather than a simple formula. The patient has clearly assimilated some of the education which gives her control: she understands that good glucose control is important, that blood glucose levels are modifiable by insulin, and that a short-acting insulin will control a glycaemic peak of short duration. The answer offers further insights: that trends rather than possible freak events are important; that research is needed before making permanent adjustments; and that there are other options than a "knee-jerk" response. The dilemma, then, is how to share a vast amount of information, to cover all eventualities, without overwhelming and confusing the patient. One solution, of progressive education according to need, requires easy access to advice and time. In the real world, the delivery of this solution is haphazard, prolonged and inefficent, despite our best efforts.

Do you think that complementary or alternative medicine can help people with diabetes?

Alternative medicine suggests a form of treatment that is taken in the place of conventional medical treatment. As such this could potentially be very dangerous, particularly if your diabetes is treated with insulin.

However, there may be a place for complementary therapies that can be tried alongside conventional medicine. Although there is no scientific evidence to show that complementary therapies such as yoga, reflexology, hypnosis or aromatherapy can benefit someone with diabetes, some people who have tried them report they feel more relaxed. As stress can have a detrimental effect on blood glucose it may mean that their diabetes improves as a result.

We must emphasise that these therapies should always be used in addition to, not instead of, your usual diabetic treatment. You should not alter your recommended diet or stop taking your tablets or insulin, nor would a reputable complementary practitioner suggest that you do any of these things.

Is it any surprise that people, aware that conventional Western medicine cannot offer them a cure in diabetes, look elsewhere? If complementary practitioners had a cure for diabetes, this would be widely broadcast. On the other hand perhaps there are unconventional methods of stimulating endogenous insulin secretion, so it may be reasonable to try other therapies as long as precautions are taken to avoid dangerous hyperglycaemia or prolonged periods of poor control. We are, after all, quite prepared to suggest that newly diagnosed NIDDs should attempt dietary control alone for up to three months. The evidence underpinning our strategies for diabetic care is patchy at best, so perhaps an open mind about alternatives to our therapies is wise. The key point, with which few would argue, is that monitoring of blood glucose and the readiness of the patient to abandon dangerous therapies are necessary to ensure safety. This topic is a good example of our potential as advisers in a partnership in care.

I have "brittle diabetes" and my doctor has advised me to stop working. Am I entitled to any benefits?

The term "brittle diabetes" is used rather too loosely. It is usually taken to mean someone whose blood glucose rises or falls very quickly and they may develop unexpected hypos. Many conditions may contribute to this but one of the most common factors is an inappropriate dose of insulin. Other factors which may contribute include irregular meals and lifestyle, poor injection technique and general ignorance about the problems of balancing food, exercise and insulin. Few people have such difficulty in controlling their diabetes that they have to give up work, but welfare benefits are available to people with diabetes in the same way as they are to anyone else.

If, indeed, there are solutions to this person's disabling diabetes, then he has suffered the double insult of an inaccurate diagnosis and poor advice. This patient has been invited to add a social disability to an illness management failure. His problem is his doctor. What a potential we have for inappropriately influencing people's lives as a result of our ignorance!

I have seen a programme on the television which says that human insulin may be dangerous. My 14-year-old son has just developed diabetes and I see that the doctor has put him on human insulin. You can imagine how worried I am about it.

Yes, it is unfortunate that this programme appeared at such a bad time for you. The people who make these programmes do not realise the fear and anxiety they can cause.

First you must believe that your son needs insulin – without it he would soon become very ill. It does not really matter at this stage what sort of insulin he has although most doctors in this country start people who need insulin on the human variety. The only problems with human insulin seem to be caused by the change over from pork to human insulin. As your son has been on human insulin from the start he should not run into any difficulties. Perhaps you should talk to a family in which one of the children has had diabetes for a few years. They would probably be able to give the reassurance you need.

Our patients may have a keener nose for information about their condition than we. This parent's "dilemma" was the duty of care for a child threatened by new and worrying information. As doctors, when we watch any television programme about medicine, we are reminded not to trust a single detail. The best broadcasters still don't know the difference between a virus and a bacterium. On the other hand, the makers of television programmes are communicators of exceptional talent. They would be failing in their calling if they couldn't instil this sort of worry in the non-medical public.

Should I warn fellow employees that I may be subject to hypos?

Definitely. Hypos unfortunately can happen, especially when a person first starts using insulin. Warn your workmates that if they find you acting in a peculiar way they must get you to take some sugar. Warn them also that you may not be very co-operative at the time and even resist their attempts to help you. Some people find it difficult to admit to their colleagues that they have diabetes, but if you keep it a secret you run the risk of causing a scare by having a bad hypo and being taken to hospital by ambulance for treatment. A needless trip to hospital should be avoided.

This is a common problem, a conflict between embarrassment and safety. It revolves around anxiety that there is a stigma attached to diabetes, so evidence of diabetes such as a hypo becomes embarrassing. This may become a "self-fulfilling prophecy". The advice given should go some way to destigmatising the condition. An additional ploy might be to ask the patient how, if he did not have diabetes, he would react to a colleague at work with diabetes who had a hypo, and then suggest his workmates would show the same generosity and concern.

I am 18 and go out a lot with my friends. I am careful never to drink and drive but when it is not my turn to drive I do drink quite a lot. I am careful not to miss any meals and I am not increasing my insulin as I used to when I first started drinking but I have had quite a few bad hypos recently. Why should this happen?

Briefly, because alcohol blocks the release of glucose from the liver. If your blood glucose is dropping because it is quite a while since you have eaten or because you have been out and active longer than usual, then your body cannot come to the rescue as it normally does. Ideally it would have been better if you could try not to have more than three or four units of alcohol in any one session. If you are going to have more than three or four units in one go, then make sure you have your usual meal before you go out, have a snack while out and, very importantly, have a sandwich or a take-away meal before you go to bed. Following this plan will help prevent your hypos.

Here, the dilemma lies between the young person's wish to be like his friends and the constraints of diabetes. What a delightful response this is. It combines education directed at an expressed need with acceptance of less than ideal behaviour (as may well be the case in the real world) and sound advice for this eventuality. The health adviser will probably earn a lot of respect which will be useful in the future.

My husband, who is middle aged with insulin dependent diabetes, has been impotent for the past two years. Please will you explain his condition as I am worried that my teenage son, who also has diabetes, may also discover that he is impotent.

Impotence (or the fear of it) worries many people and is certainly not so rare that we can ignore it. It has been claimed that as many as 20% of males with diabetes (though the figure is probably not as high as this) may at some stage become impotent. Most impotent men are not suffering from diabetes: anxiety, depression, overwork, tiredness, stress, guilt, alcohol excess and grief can contribute to impotence. Any man may find that he is temporarily impotent and there is no reason why men with diabetes should not experience this. Fear of failure can perpetuate the condition. Overwork or worry is frequently the cause of lack of interest in sex and even of impotence. Excess alcohol can cause prolonged lack of potency.

Some men with diabetes do become impotent, due to problems with the blood supply or the nerve supply to the penis. This usually develops slowly and in the younger person we believe it can be prevented by strict blood glucose control. In the older person (who does not require insulin) the condition does not usually respond well to treatment. In this age group impotence is more commonly due to other factors and not to diabetes. We hope you will be encouraged to discuss the matter further with your own doctor or with the doctor at the diabetes clinic which your husband and son attend.

This woman is quite explicit. She wants to know about "impotence" so that she can counsel her son, should he discover Dad's problem. But is there a hidden agenda? Does she want to know about treatment options? How is she managing? The possibility of erectile failure is a worry to men in a our society and that worry extends to discussing the subject. One has only to recall the opening remarks of so many patients in this context: "you will think it is a bit silly to be worrying about this at my age", or "I have a delicate matter to raise", for example, to confirm the difficulty men may have in broaching the topic. Perhaps we should routinely ask about erectile failure as we do about hypos, in order to open doors for discussion both now and in the future.

My 15 year old son developed diabetes at the age of 12. Initially he was very sensible about his diabetes but recently he has become resentful, saying he is different from everyone else and blaming us for his disease. What do you suggest?

You must first realise that most people of all ages (and their parents) feel resentful at some stage about this disease which causes so much inconvenience in someone's life. Many 12 year old children conform with their parents wishes and generally do as they are told. However, by the age of 15 other important pressures are beginning to bear on a developing young person. In the case of a boy, the most important factors in life are (1) his friends and (2) girls. While you as parents are prepared to make allowances and provide special meals etc., most young lads want to join the gang and do not wish to appear "different".

At a Firbush camp (which was restricted to hand-picked, well-adjusted young adults with diabetes), the organisers were horrified to discover how angry young people felt about their condition. Of course this anger will often be directed at the parents. We can only give advice in general terms which apply to most adolescent problems.

- *Keep lines of communication open*
- *Boost his self-esteem by giving praise where praise is due even if your own self-esteem is taking a hammering*
- *Allow your son to make his own decisions about diabetes. If you force him to comply, he will simply avoid confrontation by deceiving you*
- *Remember that difficult adolescents usually turn into successful adults*

The conflict here is between parental responsibility and youth in revolt. Adolescence is alleged to be difficult for everyone. It is possible that toeing the line during the teenage years, while being well received by adults, is actually abnormal and may presage some emotional problems in later life.

Understanding the variants of adolescent behaviour, however, is not helpful when the carer feels a duty of care which is being frustrated. This problem illustrates neatly how empowering patients, allowing them to become partners in care, can help both carer and patient; less guilt for the carer and an adult role for the patient. It is just as well that in adolescence parents are around to mop up the results of some of those "adult" decisions.

EDUCATION AND TRAINING OPPORTUNITIES

19

HANDLING ILLNESS

It takes two to tango. The illness may affect the patient but the doctor or nurse is involved too and can also be affected. In turn, we influence future consultations. The danger is to operate as though we have "Read Only Memories", novel episodes serving merely to confirm prejudices. In an ideal world, we would learn from every interaction and in so doing approach new ones with an open mind.

One of the attractions of general practice is the opportunity to see how patients one has known for many years respond to acute and chronic illnesses. Often, one has developed an idea of their personality which one assumes will predict how they respond to life's surprises. On reflection, one might see how earlier experiences and the coping strategies then used, in conjunction with manipulation of current information set against a background of the pressures of the time, might help to explain a particular behaviour.

Part of the fascination of medicine lies in how often our expectations are confounded. Perhaps for want of a key element in the background or ignorance of a major current stress, we may get off on completely the wrong foot. An early error, weighted by association with a significant new problem, then becomes hard to undo. Thus, the exhortation of the teachers of consultation skills to explore patients' ideas, fears and understanding may be seen to be more than simple adherence to the party line, an act of blind faith undertaken by the new doctor. It is a more certain route to an effective partnership with the patient in the joint management of a new illness.

We might assume that diabetes represents a chronic illness with profound effects on daily living and a probability of morbidity. We may, aware of the effects of lifestyle on morbidity, assume that as logic dictates a radical change so the patient will follow suit. Were he or she not to do this, we might be somewhat dismissive. Our hitherto logical, sensible patient could be a "controller" who has suddenly found the meaning of chaos and reacted by ignoring disorder and the appropriate behaviours for managing it. On the other hand, with the memory of a major morbid event recently embossed on our memories, we may assume that the patient is frightened witless by the possibility of a similar disaster and, in an effort to protect, play down the potential problems, we may convey a falsely optimistic message.

We need to understand the range of reactions of patients and know the likelihood of complications. Responses to diagnosis may be likened to spokes on a wheel with many opposites – the extremes of the elements of what might be termed a desirable reaction. Contrasting pairs on this wheel include anxious/optimistic, passive/enquiring, denial/resignation, anger/emotional emptiness, child/parent, disorganised/obsessional. The challenge for us is to identify the position and bring the patient towards the centre of the wheel using time, education and counselling. At the same time, we should be aware of our own characteristics and how they might hinder the patient in his or her centripetal journey. It is difficult, for example, for an obsessional to manage a totally disorganised person, and acting as "parent" to the "child" hinders rather than helps.

CARERS AND EDUCATION

It is important not to overlook the concerns of the partner or parent for, like as not, they are patients too and their reactions and involvement influence those of the person with diabetes. Explaining a problem to the carer not only underlines recognition of his or her role, but can result in patients learning more than they would if the education were directed at them. The carer and patient will almost certainly compare notes, thereby reinforcing the learning process.

Breaking the bad news

Above all, this takes time. The diagnosis of diabetes is shocking to most people, and with shock comes difficulty in ingesting information. We have already indicated the role of the specialist diabetes nurse in providing information over time, and we have described the grieving for loss of health and independence. An understanding of how the patient *might* feel, enquiry about how the patient *does* feel, respect and a gentle pace will go a long way towards breaking the bad news with least pain.

Getting the message across

A style appropriate to the patient, in a language devoid of jargon, with frequent checking of understanding, is a good start. Mary MacKinnon, in her practical book *Providing Diabetes Care in General Practice* lists the six common faults of information giving as perceived by the patients. They are:

- Incorrect information
- Inconsistent information
- Too much information
- Too little information

■ Inappropriate information
■ Outdated information

The synthesis

So now our patient has the perfect introduction to diabetes and is well informed. The bad news is that being well informed does not always equate with being well controlled. Such is life and the right to make choices. Such is diabetes in the real world.

THE ST VINCENT DECLARATION

The St Vincent Declaration implementation document provides guidelines for people with diabetes. These guidelines are reflected in the British Diabetic Association leaflet 'Diabetes care – what you should expect', available free on request from the British Diabetic Association, 10 Queen Anne Street, London W1, telephone 0171 323 1531.

FOR ALL PEOPLE WITH DIABETES

Your guide to better diabetes care: rights and roles

A person with diabetes can, in general, lead a normal healthy and long life. Looking after yourself (self-care) by learning about your diabetes provides the best chance to do this. Your doctor and other members of the health care team are there to advise you and to provide the information, support and technology so that you can look after yourself and live your life in the way you choose.

It is important that you know:

1. What should be available from your health care providers to help you achieve these goals
2. What *you* should do

Your rights

The health care team (providers) should provide:

■ A treatment plan and self-care targets
■ Regular checks of blood sugar (glucose) levels
■ Regular checks of your physical condition
■ Treatment for special problems and emergencies
■ Continuing education for you and your family
■ Information on available social and economic support

Your role is

■ To build this advice into your daily life
■ To be in control of your diabetes on a day to day basis

Continuing education

The following are important items you should learn about:

1. Why to control blood glucose levels
2. How to control your blood glucose levels through proper eating, physical activity, tablets and/or insulin
3. How to monitor your control with blood or urine test (self-monitoring) and how to act on the results
4. The signs of low and high blood glucose levels and ketosis, how to treat these conditions and how to prevent them
5. What to do when you are ill
6. The possible long term complications – including possible damage to eyes, nerves, kidneys and feet and hardening of the arteries; their prevention and treatment
7. How to deal with lifestyle variations such as exercise, travelling and social activities, including drinking alcohol
8. How to handle possible problems with employment, insurance, driving licences, etc. (see Note at end)

Treatment plan and self-care targets

The following should be given to you:

1. Personalised advice on proper eating – types of food, amounts and timing
2. Advice on physical activity
3. Your dose and timing of tablets or insulin and how to take them; advice on how to change doses based on your self-monitoring
4. Your target values for blood glucose, blood fats, blood pressure and weight

Regular assessment

The following should be done at each visit to your health care professionals. (NB These may vary according to your particular needs.)

1. Review of your self-monitoring results and current treatment
2. Talk about your targets and change where necessary
3. Talk about any problems and questions you may have
4. Continued education

The health care team should check the following:

1. Your blood glucose control by taking special blood tests such as those for glycosylated haemoglobin, fructosamine or fasting blood glucose in non-insulin treated people. These can be done two to four times a year if your diabetes is well controlled
2. Your weight
3. Your blood pressure and blood fats if necessary

The following should be checked at least once per year:

1. Your vision and eyes (with dilated pupils)
2. Your kidney function (blood and urine tests)
3. Your feet
4. Your risk factors for heart disease, such as blood pressure, blood fats and smoking habits
5. Your self-monitoring and injection techniques
6. Your eating habits

Special problems

1. Advice and care should be available if you are planning to become pregnant.
2. The needs of children and adolescents should be cared for
3. If you have problems with eyes, kidneys, feet, blood vessels or heart you should be able to see specialists quickly
4. In the elderly strict treatment is often unnecessary; you may want to discuss this with your health care team
5. The first months after your diabetes has been discovered are often difficult. Remember you cannot learn everything during this period – learning will continue for the rest of your life

Your role

■ Take control of your diabetes on a day to day basis. This will become easier the more you know about diabetes
■ Learn about and practise self-care. This includes monitoring glucose levels and learning how to change your treatment according to the results
■ Examine your feet regularly

- Follow good lifestyle practices. These include choosing the right food, weight control, regular physical activity and not smoking
- Know when to contact your health care team urgently, especially in an emergency
- Talk regularly with the health care team about your questions and concerns
- Ask questions and repeat them if you are still unclear. Prepare your questions beforehand
- Speak to your health care team, other people with diabetes and your local or national diabetes associations and read pamphlets and books about diabetes, provided by your health care team or diabetes association
- Make sure your family and friends know about the needs of your diabetes
- If you feel that adequate facilities and care are not available to help you look after your diabetes, contact your local or national diabetes association

Note

"The St Vincent Declaration seeks to promote independence, equity and self-sufficiency for people with diabetes and the removal of hindrances to their full integration into society."

For example:

Driving licences

"Prejudice should not prevent diabetic people whose disease is well controlled and who have satisfactory vision from driving cars or certain other types of vehicle. Steps should be taken to remove any unreasonable restrictions."

Employment

"Nearly all people with diabetes are capable of working as well as their non-diabetic fellows. Exceptions to this rule are very few. Steps should be taken to remove ignorance and prejudice in this area."

Insurance

"Although the position has improved considerably in Denmark, France, Italy and the United Kingdom, the word must be spread that diabetic people who properly monitor their disease have a near normal life expectancy and should therefore not be asked to pay heavy premiums for life or health insurance. Improvements are also needed in both motor and travel insurance."

The leaflet *Your guide to better diabetes care: rights and roles* is available from Boehringer Mannheim UK (see Appendix 3)

CHILDREN AND ADOLESCENTS

These are the St Vincent Declaration recommendations for the care of children and adolescents with diabetes.

Diagnosis

"Early symptoms of diabetes in children and adolescents (such as thirst, increased urine production and weight loss) should be made familiar not only to all health care professionals but also to the general population. Information about diabetes should be spread through the mass media and included in school curricula. Test materials for the measurement of glucose in urine should be available to all health care professionals."

Treatment

"Newly diagnosed patients should be treated at units whose staff have specialised knowledge of diabetes in children and adolescents. The diabetes care team should include a paediatric diabetologist, a dietitian, a specialist diabetes nurse and a social worker or psychologist.

"Long term care should be managed by a paediatrician experienced in the care of diabetic children. The interval between follow up visits should be one to three months, but shorter when needed: for example after major treatment adjustments. Long term glucose control should be estimated by measurement of glycosylated haemoglobin at least every three months. Growth and pubertal development should be followed regularly and values plotted on growth charts. The general practitioner can handle some acute problems and under exceptional circumstances intermediate consultation but always in consultation with the responsible diabetologist."

Recommendations

Recommendations are made for a standard of care for children and adolescents. They include education appropriate to age and including the family, school or college. This education should be provided orally and in writing and should encompass information about weekends, holidays and camps.

Recommendations for specialist teams also include:

- Psychological/social support
- Insulin treatment
- Nutrition
- Self-management
- Blood glucose control – targets
- Late vascular complications
- Social rights

PATIENT-FRIENDLY GLOSSARY

This glossary was developed for the popular book *Diabetes at Your Fingertips*, with the information needs of patients in mind. It has, however, been modified slightly to take account of differences in content and terminology used in this book. Some of the definitions may appear over simplistic unless you remember that they are aimed not at you but at someone who may have no medical knowledge at all.

The glossary is reproduced by kind permission of the authors of *Diabetes at Your Fingertips*, Peter Sönksen, Sue Judd and Charles Fox.

Terms in *italics* in these definitions refer to other terms in the glossary.

acarbose A drug which slows the digestion and absorption of complex *carbohydrates*.

Acesulfane-K A low-calorie intense sweetener.

acetone One of the chemicals called *ketones* formed when the body uses up fat for energy. The presence of acetone in the urine usually means that more insulin is needed.

adrenaline A hormone produced by the adrenal glands which prepares the body for action (the "flight or fight" reaction) and also causes an increase in blood glucose levels. Produced by the body when the blood glucose falls too low.

albumin A protein present in most animal tissues. The presence of albumin in the urine may denote a kidney or bladder infection or early kidney damage.

alpha cell The cell that produces glucagon – found in the *islets of Langerhans* in the *pancreas*.

antigens Protein substances which the body recognises as "foreign" and which trigger an immune response.

arteriosclerosis or **arterial sclerosis** or **arterial disease** Hardening of the arteries. Loss of elasticity in the walls of the arteries due to thickening and calcification. Occurs with advancing years in those with or without diabetes. May affect the heart, causing thrombosis, or affect the circulation, particularly in the legs and feet.

aspartame A low-calorie intense sweetener. Brand name NutraSweet.

autonomic neuropathy Damage to the system of nerves which regulate many autonomic functions of the body such as stomach emptying, sexual function (potency) and blood pressure control.

bacteria Germs.

balanitis Inflammation of the end of the penis, usually caused by the presence of sugar in the urine.

beef insulin Insulin extracted from the *pancreas* of cattle.

beta blockers Drugs which block the effect of stress hormones on the cardiovascular system. Often used to treat angina and to lower blood pressure. Change the warning signs of *hypoglycaemia*.

beta cell The cell which produces insulin – found in the *islets of Langerhans* in the *pancreas*.

biguanides A group of anti-diabetes tablets which lower blood glucose levels. They work by increasing the uptake of glucose by muscle, by reducing the absorption of glucose by the intestine and by reducing the amount of glucose produced by the liver. The only used preparation is metformin.

blood glucose monitoring System of measuring blood glucose levels at home using special reagent sticks or a special meter.

bran Indigestible husk of the wheat grain. A type of *dietary fibre*.

brittle diabetes Term used to refer to diabetes which is very unstable with swings from very low to very high blood glucose levels.

calories Units in which energy or heat are measured. The energy value of food is measured in calories.

carbohydrates A class of food which comprises starches and sugars and is most readily available by the body for energy. Found mainly in plant foods. Examples are rice, bread, potatoes, pasta, dried beans.

cataract Opacity of the lens of the eye which obscures vision. It may be removed surgically.

CHD Abbreviation for *coronary heart disease*.

clear insulin Soluble or regular insulin.

cloudy insulin Longer-acting insulin with fine particles of protamine or zinc.

coma A form of unconsiousness from which people can only be roused with difficulty. If caused by diabetes, may be a *diabetic coma* or an *insulin coma*.

complications Long-term consequences of imperfectly controlled diabetes.

control Usually refers to blood glucose control. The aim of good control is to achieve normal blood glucose levels (4–7 mmol/l).

coronary heart disease Disease of the blood vessels supplying the heart.

cystitis Inflammation of the bladder causing frequency of passing urine and a burning sensation when passing urine.

Dextrosol Glucose tablets.

diabetes insipidus A disorder of the pituitary gland accompanied by excessive urination and thirst.

diabetes mellitus A disorder of the *pancreas* characterised by a high blood glucose level. This book is about diabetes mellitus.

diabetic amyotrophy Rare condition causing pain and/or weakness of the legs due to the damage to certain nerves.

diabetic coma Extreme form of *hyperglycaemia*, usually with *ketoacidosis*, causing unconsciousness.

diabetic foods Food products targeted at people with diabetes, in which ordinary sugar (*sucrose*) is replaced with substitutes such as *fructose* or *sorbitol*. Not recommended as part of your food plan.

diabetic nephropathy Type of *nephropathy* which may occur in diabetes.

diabetic neuropathy Type of *neuropathy* which may occur in diabetes.

diabetic retinopathy Type of *retinopathy* which may occur in diabetes.

dietary fibre Part of plant material which resists digestion and gives bulk to the diet. Also called fibre or roughage.

diuretics Agents which increase the flow of urine, usually called water tablets.

epidural Usually referring to the type of anaesthetic that is commonly used in obstetrics. Anaesthetic solution is injected through the spinal canal to numb the lower part of the body.

exchanges Portions of *carbohydrate* foods in the diabetes diet which can be exchanged for one another. 1 exchange = 10 g carbohydrate.

fibre Another name for *dietary fibre*.

free foods Foods which contain so little *carbohydrate* that people with diabetes may have liberal helpings of them without counting them in their diet. Examples include cabbage, rhubarb, lettuce, cauliflower, tea or coffee without milk.

fructosamine Measurement of diabetes *control* which reflects the average blood glucose level over the previous two to three weeks. Similar to *haemoglobin* which averages the blood glucose over the longer period of two to three months.

fructose Type of sugar found naturally in fruit and honey. Since it does not require insulin for its *metabolism*, it is often used as a sweetener in *diabetic foods*.

gangrene Death of a part of the body due to a very poor blood supply. A combination of *neuropathy* and *arteriosclerosis* may result in infection of unrecognised injuries to the feet. If neglected this infection may spread, causing further destruction.

gene Unit of heredity controlling a particular inherited characteristic of an individual.

gestational diabetes Diabetes occurring during pregnancy.

glaucoma Disease of the eye causing increased pressure inside the eyeball.

glucagon A *hormone* produced by the *alpha cells* in the *pancreas* which causes a rise in blood glucose by freeing *glycogen* from the liver. Available in injection form and can be used to treat a severe *hypo*.

glucose Form of sugar made by digestion of *carbohydrates*. Absorbed into the blood stream where it circulates and is used for energy.

glucose tolerance test Test used in the diagnosis of *diabetes mellitus*. The glucose in the blood is measured at intervals before and after the person has drunk a large amount of glucose whilst fasting.

glycogen The form in which *carbohydrate* is stored in the liver. It is often known as animal starch.

glycosuria Presence of glucose in the urine.

glycosylated haemoglobin Another name for *haemoglobin* A1

guar A good source of dietary fibre obtainable from the cluster bean.

haemoglobin A1 The part of the haemoglobin or colouring matter of the red blood cell which has glucose attached to it. A test of diabetes *control*. The amount of haemoglobin A1 in the blood depends on the average blood glucose level over the previous two to three months.

honeymoon period Time when the dose of insulin drops shortly after starting insulin treatment. It is the result of partial recovery of insulin secretion by the *pancreas*. Usually the honeymoon period only lasts for a short time.

hormone Substance generated in one gland or organ which is carried by the blood to another part of the body to stimulate another organ into activity. *Insulin* and *glucagon* are both hormones.

human insulin Insulin which has been manufactured to be identical to that produced in the human *pancreas*. Differs slightly from older insulins which were extracted from cows or pigs.

hydramnios An excessive amount of amniotic fluid, i.e. the fluid surrounding the fetus.

hyperglycaemia High blood glucose (above 10 mmol/l).

hyperlipidaemia An excess of fats (or lipids) in the blood.

hypo Abbreviation for *hypoglycaemia*.

hypoglycaemia (also known as a hypo or an insulin reaction) Low blood glucose (below 3 mmol/l).

IDD Abbreviation for insulin dependent diabetic.

IDDM Abbreviation for *insulin dependent diabetes mellitus*.

impotence Failure of erection of the penis.

injector Device to aid injections.

insulin A *hormone* produced by the *beta cells* of the *pancreas* and responsible for the control of blood glucose. Insulin can only be given by injection because digestive juices destroy its action if taken by mouth.

insulin coma Extreme form of *hypoglycaemia* associated with unconsciousness and sometimes convulsions.

insulin dependent diabetes mellitus (abbreviation IDDM) Type of diabetes which cannot be treated without insulin. Most common in younger people and is also called *type I diabetes* or *juvenile-onset diabetes*.

insulin pen Device that resembles a large fountain pen that takes a cartridge of insulin. The injection of insulin is given after dialling the dose and pressing a button that releases the insulin.

insulin reaction Another name for *hypoglycaemia* or a hypo. In America it is called an insulin shock or shock.

intermediate-acting insulin Insulin preparations with action lasting 12 to 18 hours.

intradermal Meaning 'into the skin'. Usually refers to an injection given into the most superficial layer of the skin. Insulin must not be given in this way as it is painful and will not be absorbed properly.

intramuscular A deep injection into the muscle.

islets of Langerhans Specialised cells within the *pancreas* that produce *insulin* and *glucagon*.

isophane A form of *intermediate-acting insulin* which has protamine added to slow its absorption.

joule Unit of work or energy used in the metric system. About 4.18 joules in each *calorie*. Some dietitians calculate food energy in joules.

juvenile-onset diabetes Outdated name for *insulin dependent diabetes*, so called because most patients receiving insulin develop diabetes under the age of 40. The term is no longer used because insulin dependent diabetes can occur at any age.

ketoacidosis A serious condition due to lack of insulin which results in body fat being used up to form *ketones* and acids. Characterised by high blood glucose levels, ketones in the urine, vomiting, drowsiness, heavy laboured breathing and a smell of acetone on the breath.

ketones Acid substances formed when body fat is used up to provide energy.

ketonuria The presence of *acetone* and other *ketones* in the urine. Detected by testing with a special testing stick (Ketostix, Ketur Test) or tablet (Acetest). Presence of ketones in the urine is due to lack of insulin or periods of starvation.

laser treatment Process in which laser beams are used to treat a damaged retina (back of the eye). Used in *photocoagulation*.

lente insulin A form of *intermediate-acting insulin* which has zinc added to slow its absorption.

lipoatrophy Loss of fat from injection sites. It used to occur before the use of highly purified insulins.

lipohypertrophy Fatty swelling usually caused by repeated injections of insulin into the same site.

maturity onset diabetes Another term for non-insulin dependent diabetes most commonly occurring in people who are middle-aged and overweight. Also called type II diabetes.

metabolic rate Rate of oxygen consumption by the body, rate at which you "burn up" the food you eat.

metabolism Process by which the body turns food into energy.

microaneurysms Small red dots on the *retina* at the back of the eye which are one of the earliest signs of diabetic *retinopathy*. Represent areas of weakness of the very small blood vessels in the eye. Microaneurysms do not affect the eyesight in any way.

micromole One thousandth (1/1000) of a *millimole*.

millimole Unit for measuring the concentration of glucose and other substances in the blood. Blood glucose is measured in millimoles per litre (mmol/l). It has replaced milligrams per decilitre (mg/dl or mg%) as a unit of measurement although this is still used in some other countries. 1 mmol/l = 18 mg/dl.

nephropathy Kidney damage. In the first instance this makes the kidney more leaky so that *albumin* appears in the urine. At a later stage it may affect the function of the kidney and in severe cases lead to kidney failure.

neuropathy Damage to the nerves, which may be *peripheral neuropathy* or *autonomic neuropathy*. It can occur with diabetes especially when poorly controlled, but also has other causes.

NIDD Abbreviation for non-insulin dependent diabetic.

NIDDM Abbreviation for *non-insulin dependent diabetes mellitus*.

non-insulin dependent diabetes mellitus (abbreviation NIDDM) Type of diabetes which occurs in older people who are often overweight. These people do not always need insulin treatment and usually can be successfully controlled with diet alone or diet and tablets. Also known as type II or maturity-onset diabetes.

pancreas Gland lying behind the stomach which as well as secreting a digestive fluid (pancreatic juice) also produces the hormone *insulin*. Contains *islets of Langerhans*.

peripheral neuropathy Damage to the nerves supplying the muscles and skin. This can result in diminished sensation, particularly in the feet and legs, and in muscle weakness.

phimosis Inflammation and narrowing of the foreskin of the penis.

photocoagulation Process of treating diabetic *retinopathy* with light beams, either laser beams or xenon arc. This technique focuses a beam of light on a very tiny area of the *retina*. This beam is so intense that it causes a very small burn, which may close off a leaking blood vessel or destroy weak blood vessels which are likely to bleed.

polydipsia Being excessively thirsty and drinking too much. It is a symptom of untreated diabetes.

polyuria The passing of large quantities of urine due to excess glucose from the blood stream. It is a symptom of untreated diabetes.

pork insulin Insulin extracted from the *pancreas* of pigs.

protein One of the classes of food that is necessary for growth and repair of tissues. Found in fish, meat, eggs, milk and pulses. Can also refer to albumin when found in the urine.

proteinuria Protein or *albumin* in the urine.

pruritus vulvae Irritation of the vulva (the genital area in women). Caused by an infection that occurs because of an excess of sugar in the urine and is often an early sign of diabetes in the older person. It clears up when the blood glucose levels return to normal and the sugar disappears from the urine.

pulses Peas, beans and lentils.

pyelonephritis Inflammation and infection of the kidney.

renal threshold The level of glucose in the blood above which it will begin to spill into the urine. The usual renal threshold for glucose in the blood is about 10 mmol/l, i.e. when the blood glucose rises above 10 mmol/l, glucose appears in the urine.

retina Light-sensitive coat at the back of the eye.

retinopathy Damage to the *retina*.

roughage Another name for *dietary fibre*.

saccharin A synthetic sweetener which is calorie-free.

short-acting insulin Insulin preparations with action lasting 6 to 12 hours.

Snellen chart Chart showing rows of letters in decreasing sizes. Used for measuring *visual acuity*.

sorbitol A chemical related to sugar and alcohol which is used as a sweetening agent in foods as a substitute for ordinary sugar. It has no significant effect upon the blood glucose level but has the same number of calories as ordinary sugar so should not be used by those who need to lose weight. Poorly absorbed and may have a laxative effect.

steroids Hormones produced by the adrenal glands, testes and ovaries. Also available in synthetic form.

subcutaneous injection An injection beneath the skin into the layer of fat which lies between the skin and muscle.

sucrose A sugar (containing *glucose* and *fructose* in combination) derived from sugar cane or sugar beet (i.e. ordinary table sugar). It has a high carbohydrate and calorie content.

sulphonylureas Anti-diabetes tablets which lower the blood glucose by stimulating the *pancreas* to produce more insulin. Commonly used sulphonylureas are glibenclamide and chlorpropamide.

syndrome X A cluster of medical problems: diabetes, hypertension, central obesity, abnormal lipids.

thrombosis Clot forming in a blood vessel.

tissue markers Proteins on the outside of cells in the body which are genetically determined.

toxaemia Poisoning of the blood by the absorption of toxins. Usually refers to the toxaemia of pregnancy which is characterised by high blood pressure, *proteinuria* and ankle swelling.

type I diabetes Another name for *insulin dependent diabetes*. Age of onset is usually below the age of 40 years.

type II diabetes Another name for *non-insulin dependent diabetes*.

Age of onset is usually above the age of 40 years.

U40 insulin The old weaker strength of insulin, no longer available in the UK. It is still the standard insulin in many European countries.

U100 insulin The standard strength of insulin in the UK, USA, Canada, Australia, New Zealand, South Africa, the Middle East and the Far East.

urine testing The detection of abnormal amounts of *glucose*, *ketones*, *protein* or blood in the urine, usually by means of urine testing sticks.

virus A very small organism capable of causing disease.

viscous fibre A type of *dietary fibre* found in *pulses* (peas, beans and lentils) and some fruit and vegetables.

visual acuity Acuteness of vision. Measured by reading letters on a sight testing chart (a *Snellen chart*).

water tablets The common name for *diuretics*.

RESOURCES

USEFUL ADDRESSES

British Diabetic Association
10 Queen Anne Street, London W1M 0BD
Tel: 0171 323 1531

British Diabetic Association (Publications)
PO Box 1, Portishead, Bristol BS20 8DJ
Tel: 01275 818700

British Dietetic Association
7th Floor, Elizabeth House, 22 Suffolk Street Queensway,
    Birmingham B1 1LS
Tel: 0121 643 5483

British Heart Foundation
41 Fitzhardinge Street, London W1 4DH
Tel: 0171 935 0185

Disability Alliance
Universal House, Wentworth Street, London E1 7SA
Tel: 0171 247 8776

Manchester Diabetes Centre (Mrs Sue Higgins)
130 Hathersage Road, Manchester M13 0HZ
Tel: 0161 276 6700

National Kidney Federation
6 Stanley Street, Worksop, Nottinghamshire S81 7HX
Tel: 01909 487795

Outward Bound Eskdale
Eskdale Green, Holmbrook, Cumbria CA19 1TE
Tel: 019467 23281

Royal National Institute for the Blind
224 Great Portland Street London W1N 6AA
Tel: 0171 388 1266

Support After Termination for Fetal Abnormality (SAFTA)
73-75 Charlotte Street, London W1P 1LB
Tel: 0171 631 0280; Patient helpline 0171 631 0285

LIFE INSURANCE AND PENSIONS

For information about BDA Insurance Services, send for a copy
of the leaflet 'Diabetes and Insurance'.

BDA Motor Quoteline Tel: 01903 262900

BDA Life Assurance Quoteline Tel: 0161 829 5600

BDA Travel Quoteline Tel: 0171 512 0890

COMPANIES

Bayer Diagnostics
Bayer plc, Evans House, Hamilton Close, Basingstoke,
  Hampshire RG21 2YE
Tel: 01256 29181

Becton Dickinson UK Ltd
Between Towns Road, Cowley, Oxford OX4 3LY
Tel: 01865 748844

Boehringer Mannheim UK (BM)
Rapid Diagnostics Division, Bell Lane, Lewes, East Sussex
BN7 1LG
Tel: 01273 480444

CP Pharmaceuticals
North Wrexham Industrial Estate, Wrexham, Clwyd LL13 9UF
Tel: 01978 661262

Hypoguard UK Ltd
Dock Lane, Melton Woodridge, Suffolk IP12 1PE
Tel: 01394 387333/4

LifeScan / Ortho Diagnostics
Enterprise House, Station Road, Loudwater, High Wycombe
HP10 9UF
Tel: 01494 442211

Lilly Diabetes Care Division
Dextra Court, Chapel Hill, Basingstoke, Hampshire
Tel: 01256 473241

Lipha Pharmaceuticals Ltd,
Harrier House, High Street, Yiewsley, West Drayton,
Middlesex UB7 7QG
Tel: 01895 449331

Medic-Alert Foundation
17 Bridge Wharf, 156 Caledonian Road, London N1 9UU
Tel: 0171 833 3034

MediSense Britain Ltd
PO Box 20159, Coleshill, Birmingham B46 1HZ
Tel: 01675 467044

Novo Nordisk Pharmaceuticals Ltd
Novo Nordisk House, Broadfield Park, Brighton Road, Pease
Pottage, Crawley, West Sussex RH11 9RT
Tel: 01293 613555

Nycomed (UK) Ltd
2111 Coventry Road, Sheldon, Birmingham B26 3EA
Tel: 0121 742 2444

Owen Mumford Ltd (Medical shop)
Brook Hill, Woodstock, Oxford OX7 1TU
Tel: 01993 812021

Pharmacia Ltd
Davy Avenue, Knowlhi Hill, Milton Keynes MK5 8PH
Tel: 01908 661101

Servier Laboratories Ltd
Metabolic Division, Fulmer Hall, Windmill Road, Fulmer,
   Slough, Buckinghamshire SL3 6HH
Tel: 01753 662744

SOS/Talisman
Golden Key Co Ltd, 1 Hare Street, Sheerness, Kent ME12 1AH
Tel: 01795 663403

3M Health Care Ltd
3M House, Morley Street, Loughborough, Leicestershire
   LE11 0BR
Tel: 01509 611611

JOURNALS

For professionals
Diabetes Care, four issues per year available from:
   Colwood House Medical Publications (UK) Ltd, Kirtons
   Farm, Pingewood, Reading, Berkshire RG3 3UN
Diabetes in General Practice, four issues per year available from:
   PMH Publications International, PO Box 100, Chichester,
   West Sussex PO18 8HD
Diabetic Medicine, ten issues per year available from:
   John Wiley and Sons Ltd, Baffins Lane, Chichester, West
   Sussex PO19 1UD

Diabetes Update, two issues per year (free) available from the British Diabetic Association

Practical Diabetes, six issues per year available from:
PMH Publications International, PO Box 100, Chichester, West Sussex PO18 8HD

For patients

Balance, six issues a year (free) available from the British Diabetic Association

Balance for Beginners: Insulin dependent diabetes

Balance for Beginners: Non-insulin dependent diabetes
— both available from the British Diabetic Association

BOOKS

For professionals

Alberti KGMM, DeFronzo RA, Keen H, Zimmet P (1992) *International textbook of diabetes mellitus*. John Wiley & Sons, Chichester

European NIDDM Policy Group (1993) *A desktop guide for the management of non- insulin dependent diabetes mellitus* (NIDDM), 2nd edn. Boehringer Mannheim, Germany

MacKinnon M (1995) *Providing diabetes care in general practice*, 2nd edn. CLASS Publishing, London

Pickup J, Williams G (191) *Textbook of diabetes*. Blackwell Science, Oxford

Tattersall R, Gale E (1990) *Diabetes: clinical management*. Longman, Harlow

Waine C (1992) *Diabetes (in general practice)*, 3rd edn. RCGP, London

For patients/carers

Day J, Brenchley S, Redmond S (1990) *Living with non-insulin dependent diabetes*. Medikos Ltd, Sussex

Hillson R (1992) *Diabetes: a new guide*. Optima, London

Knopfler A (1992) *Diabetes and pregnancy*. Optima, London

North J (1990) *Teenage diabetes*. Thorsons, London

Sönksen P, Fox C, Judd S (1994) *Diabetes at your fingertips*, 3rd edn. CLASS Publishing, London

Many leaflets/booklets on specific topics available from the British Diabetic Association.

Contact their Publications Department (Tel: 01275 818700) for further details.

INDEX